Epidemiology

EPIDEMIOLOGY

CHARLOTTE BAKER

PDF AND EPUB FREE ONLINE AT: https://doi.org/10.21061/epidemiology

Charlotte Baker in association with the Open Education Initiative
of the University Libraries at Virginia Tech
Blacksburg, VA

Suggested citation: Baker, Charlotte (2023). *Epidemiology*. Blacksburg: Charlotte Baker. https://doi.org/10.21061/epidemiology. Licensed with CC BY-NC-SA 4.0 https://creativecommons.org/licenses/by-nc-sa/4.0.

Publisher: This work is published by Charlotte Baker in association with the Open Education Initiative of the University Libraries at Virginia Tech.

Open Education Initiative, University Libraries at Virginia Tech
560 Drillfield Drive
Blacksburg, VA 24061

Accessibility statement: Virginia Tech is committed to making its publications accessible in accordance with the Americans with Disabilities Act of 1990. The Open Education Initiative is committed to continuous improvement regarding accessibility. The text, images, and links in the PDF and ePub versions of this text are tagged structurally and include alternative text, which allows for machine readability. Please contact openeducation@vt.edu if you are a person with a disability and have suggestions to make this book more accessible.

Publication cataloging information:
Charlotte Baker
Epidemiology | Charlotte Baker
Pages cm
ISBN 978-1-957213-63-7 (PDF)
ISBN 978-1-957213-62-0 (Print)
ISBN 978-1-957213-64-4 (ePub)
ISBN 978-1-957213-65-1 (Pressbooks) https://pressbooks.lib.vt.edu/epidemiology
URI (Universal Resource Identifier): http://hdl.handle.net/10919/116257
DOI: https://doi.org/10.21061/epidemiology

Epidemiology--Textbooks.
Title: Epidemiology
RA651 .B35

Cover art: Clay Banks via https://unsplash.com/photos/cEzMOp5FtV4 | Unsplash license
Cover design and illustrations: Kindred Grey

CONTENTS

INTRODUCTION

This textbook is intended as a primer and reference for students in medical school taking an epidemiology course, preparing for the USMLE Step 1 Exam, or needing to refresh on epidemiologic concepts. Medical school students in the United States must have a basic grasp of epidemiology and how it is used in population health and clinical medicine to continue past the first year of medical school. This textbook is designed for these students and contains information that can support students as they progress in their clinical career. The goal of this textbook is to provide students with the basics of epidemiology terms and concepts.

This textbook begins with an introduction to general concepts of epidemiology, including the definition of the field, basic terms such as incidence and prevalence, and descriptions of the ways information can be counted. It progresses to how measurements and calculations in epidemiology are applied to different study designs, why one might choose a particular study design to answer a clinical question, and detailed use of measures of association and effect in different study designs. After demonstrating how epidemiology is used in clinical diagnosis and screening of disease, the textbook ends with an overview and examples of sources of error in epidemiologic studies, including bias, confounding, and effect modification.

This textbook is meant for clinical students without backgrounds in public health, particularly those who are seeking a medical degree. Ideally, students in any clinical field, including nursing and physical therapy, can use this text as a reference for epidemiologic concepts that surface while taking care of patients or learning about different conditions. This book specifically will guide medical school students as they prepare for the USMLE Step 1 Exam and to transition from student to clinician.

The author chose to write this text while teaching medical school students epidemiology. The author noticed a large gap between the detail public health students needed to know (and subsequently what most textbooks focused on) and what medical school students needed to know. No other book explained the concepts at a level simple enough to be truly introductory and appropriate for a medical school audience. This matters because these two groups of students will work together throughout their careers, but the group of medical school students have a different reason to need to know this information and how it should be used. A textbook to approach their needs was necessary.

This textbook is heavily driven by practical examples, the majority of which are sports-related. It is an open access and openly licensed textbook available digitally at no cost and features accessible text and graphics.

Parts of This Book

- Chapter 1, Epidemiology in Sum, explains the overarching idea of epidemiology.
- Chapter 2, Measuring Things in Epidemiology, explains how things are counted and the dynamics of disease.
- Chapter 3, Study Designs, includes study designs and related measures.
- Chapter 4, Diagnostics and Screening, covers the use of epidemiology in disease diagnosis and screening.
- Chapter 5, The Wrecking Ball, examines bias, confounding, interaction and effect modification, including what they are and how to work with them.
- Appendix, Study Guides, includes handwritten visual summaries of chapters 2, 3, and 4.

What Content in This Text Is Relevant to the USMLE Step 1 Exam?

The following table shows which chapters in this text are in alignment with the *First Aid for the USMLE Step 1* book (2022 edition): L. Tao, B. Vikas, and S. Matthew, *First Aid for the USMLE Step 1 2022*, 32nd ed., McGraw Hill LLC, 2022.

Chapter in this text	USMLE Step 1 material	Additional material relevant to research and clinical medicine
Chapter 1	Sections 1.1-Section 1.2	Section 1.3
Chapter 2	Sections 2.1-2.2, 2.3.1.2, 2.3.2, 2.4	Section 2.3.1.1
Chapter 3	Sections 3.1-3.6	Section 3.7
Chapter 4	Entire chapter	—
Chapter 5	Sections 5.1, 5.1.1, 5.1.2, 5.1.3, 5.2	Section 5.1.2.1

ABOUT THE AUTHOR

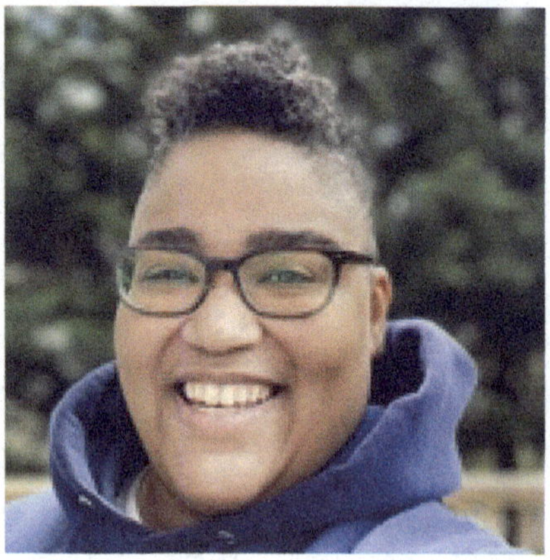

Charlotte Baker, DrPH, MPH, CPH, is the director of Epidemiology and Health Equity Lead at Truveta. She was formerly a member of the faculty in the Virginia Tech Data and Decisions Destination Area and PI of the analytic epidemiology I-SPY DATA Lab in the Department of Population Health Sciences in the Virginia-Maryland College of Veterinary Medicine. As a self-described certified data nerd, her research lab and consulting efforts prioritize bridging the methodological and data gaps in sports injury research by using advanced statistical analysis and large data sets, especially to address disparities in sport and recreation caused by social and structural determinants of health. A former epidemic intelligence service officer at the Centers for Disease Control and Prevention, her favorite use of data includes helping communities improve themselves, keeping kids safe when being physically active, and helping all of us to live our best (and healthy) lives no matter where we started.

ACKNOWLEDGMENTS

Editorial Team

Anita Walz, Managing Editor

Anita Walz is Associate Professor, Assistant Director of Open Education, and Scholarly Communication Librarian in the University Libraries at Virginia Tech. She received her MS in library and information science from the University of Illinois at Urbana-Champaign and has worked in university, government, school, and international libraries for over 20 years. She is the founder of the Open Education Initiative at Virginia Tech and the managing editor of many open textbooks adapted or created at Virginia Tech, most of which may be found by visiting https://guides.lib.vt.edu/oer. She has provided overall planning, project coordination, rights negotiation, day-to-day management, coaching, problem-solving, oversight, and post-production marketing for this book.

Kindred Grey, Illustrator, Editorial Assistant, Production Manager

Kindred Grey is the OER, Graphic Design, and Digital Publishing Specialist in the University Libraries at Virginia Tech. She joined University Libraries after receiving her B.S. in Statistics and Psychology from Virginia Tech in 2020. Kindred has contributed to over twenty open textbooks, providing technical support on layout and design. Her main focus is publishing open textbooks that are visually appealing, accessible, student oriented, and technologically advanced. She illustrated this book and also led production efforts including accessibility and formatting for the PDF, EPUB, print, and HTML versions of the text.

Special Thanks

Thank you to Dr. Eleanor Fleming and Lauren Canary for taking time out of their busy days to provide feedback on this book.

Thank you to Elly Lloyd for her careful review of this book's figures and for taking the time to ensure alternative text was provided for each one.

Publication of this work was made possible in part by a grant from the University Libraries at Virginia Tech through its Open Education Initiative (https://vtechworks.lib.vt.edu/handle/10919/70959), which provides development assistance and financial support to Virginia Tech faculty who wish to use, create, or adapt openly licensed teaching materials to support student learning.

INSTRUCTOR RESOURCES

Please use the instructor interest form if you are an instructor who is reviewing, using, or adapting *Epidemiology* for a course, or if you have created any materials related to this book and would like to share them publicly.

Navigate to the book's main landing page to access:

- Links to multiple electronic versions of the textbook (PDF, EPUB, HTML)
- A link to Amazon for ordering a print copy
- A link to the errata document
- A link to report errors

If you are interested in making your own version of this book, check out the book's license and information on best practices for attribution.

About Open Educational Resources (OER)

OER are free teaching and learning materials that are licensed to allow for revision and reuse. They can be fully self-contained textbooks, videos, quizzes, learning modules, and more. OER are distinct from free online resources in that they permit others to use, copy, distribute, modify, or reuse the content. The legal permission to modify and customize OER to meet the specific learning objectives of a particular course make them a useful pedagogical tool.

About Pressbooks

Pressbooks is an open source, web-based authoring tool based on WordPress. Virginia Tech personnel use it to create and adapt openly licensed course materials. Pressbooks offers an intuitive editing environment for educators interested in customizing this book.

About This Book

Helpful URLs

Main landing page (DOI): https://doi.org/10.21061/epidemiology

CC BY-NC-SA 4.0 license: https://creativecommons.org/licenses/by-nc-sa/4.0

Instructor interest form: https://bit.ly/interest_epidemiology

View errata: https://bit.ly/errata_epidemiology

Report an error: https://bit.ly/reporterror_epidemiology

Pressbooks (HTML): https://pressbooks.lib.vt.edu/epidemiology

Best practices for attribution: https://wiki.creativecommons.org/wiki/Best_practices_for_attribution

1. EPIDEMIOLOGY IN SUM

1.1 What Exactly Is Epidemiology?

> Epidemiology is the study of the distribution and determinants of health-related states or events (including disease) and the application of this study to the control of diseases and other health problems.
>
> —*World Health Organization*[1,2]

Epidemiology is the foundational science of public health and population health. Epidemiologic studies are applied to help control health problems in **populations**. Examples of populations are patients in a single hospital, patients seen by a particular practice, people living in a particular town or group of towns, and people with a particular disease. Epidemiology is the study of the ***distribution*** and ***determinants*** of ***health-related states or events*** (including disease) and the ***application*** of this study to the ***control* of diseases and other health problems**.[3,4] Very simply put, epidemiology is the study of how many people got sick, how they got sick, and why they got sick. For our purposes, epidemiology is important for clinical decision making (e.g., diagnostics) and for continuing education on the *who, what, where, when, why*, and *how* of health.

- ***Distribution*** – The frequency of disease occurrence. This may vary from one population group to another. An example is the "Top 10 Causes of Death in the United States,"[5] published annually by the National Center for Health Statistics,[6] a part of the Centers for Disease Control and Prevention[7] (figure 1.1).

	Age Groups										
Rank	**<1**	**1-4**	**44690**	**44848**	**15-24**	**25-34**	**35-44**	**45-54**	**55-64**	**65+**	**All Ages**
1	Congenital Anomalies 4,043	**Unintentional Injury 1,153**	**Unintentional Injury 685**	**Unintentional Injury 881**	**Unintentional Injury 15,117**	**Unintentional Injury 31,315**	**Unintentional Injury 31,057**	Malignant Neoplasms 34,589	Malignant Neoplasms 110,243	Heart Disease 556,665	Heart Disease 696,962
2	Short Gestation 3,141	Congenital Anomalies 382	Malignant Neoplasms 382	Suicide 581	Homicide 6,466	Suicide 8,454	Heart Disease 12,177	Heart Disease 34,169	Heart Disease 88,551	Malignant Neoplasms 440,753	Malignant Neoplasms 602,350
3	SIDS 1,389	Homicide 311	Congenital Anomalies 171	Malignant Neoplasms 410	Suicide 6,062	Homicide 7,125	Malignant Neoplasms 10,730	**Unintentional Injury 27,819**	COVID-19 42,090	COVID-19 282,836	COVID-19 350,831
4	**Unintentional Injury 1,194**	Malignant Neoplasms 307	Homicide 169	Homicide 285	Malignant Neoplasms 1,306	Heart Disease 3,984	Suicide 7,314	COVID-19 16,964	**Unintentional Injury 28,915**	Cerebro-vascular 137,392	**Unintentional Injury 200,955**
5	Maternal Pregnancy Comp. 1,116	Heart Disease 112	Heart Disease 56	Congenital Anomalies 150	Heart Disease 870	Malignant Neoplasms 3,573	COVID-19 6,079	Liver Disease 9,503	Chronic Low. Respiratory Disease 18,816	Alzheimer's Disease 132,741	Cerebro-vascular 160,264
6	Placenta Cord Membranes 700	Influenza & Pneumonia 84	Influenza & Pneumonia 55	Heart Disease 111	COVID-19 501	COVID-19 2,254	Liver Disease 4,938	Diabetes Mellitus 7,546	Diabetes Mellitus 18,002	Chronic Low. Respiratory Disease 128,712	Chronic Low. Respiratory Disease 152,657
7	Bacterial Sepsis 542	Cerebro-vascular 55	Chronic Low. Respiratory Disease 54	Chronic Low. Respiratory Disease 93	Congenital Anomalies 384	Liver Disease 1,631	Homicide 4,482	Suicide 7,249	Liver Disease 16,151	Diabetes Mellitus 72,194	Alzheimer's Disease 134,242
8	Respiratory Distress 388	Perinatal Period 54	Cerebro-vascular 32	Diabetes Mellitus 50	Diabetes Mellitus 312	Diabetes Mellitus 1,168	Diabetes Mellitus 2,904	Cerebro-vascular 5,686	Cerebro-vascular 14,153	**Unintentional Injury 62,796**	Diabetes Mellitus 102,188
9	Circulatory System Disease 386	Septicemia 43	Benign Neoplasms 28	Influenza & Pneumonia 50	Chronic Low. Respiratory Disease 220	Cerebro-vascular 600	Cerebro-vascular 2,008	Chronic Low. Respiratory Disease 3,538	Suicide 7,160	Nephritis 42,675	Influenza & Pneumonia 53,544
10	Neonatal Hemorrhage 317	Benign Neoplasms 35	Suicide 20	Cerebro-vascular 44	Complicated Pregnancy 191	Complicated Pregnancy 594	Influenza & Pneumonia 1,148	Homicide 2,542	Influenza & Pneumonia 6,295	Influenza & Pneumonia 42,511	Nephritis 52,547

Figure 1.1: Top 10 leading causes of death in the United States (2020).

- ***Determinants*** – Factors that are capable of bringing about change in health. Examples include things that are CBRE (chemical, biological, radiological, or explosive), environment, stress, and **social determinants of health**. (See section 1.2.)
- ***Health-related states or events*** – These include but are certainly not limited to disease, behavior, utilization of health services, drugs, and health outcomes. Examples include infectious diseases, disabilities, hospital bed capacity, life expectancy, mental health, chronic disease, and injury.
- ***Application*** – Epidemiology has its own particular measures and also applies biostatistics to identify and solve problems.
- ***Control*** – Epidemiology has four aims: to describe the health status of populations, to explain the etiology of disease, to predict the occurrence of disease, and to control the occurrence of disease. Prevention is the ultimate solution. There are three types of prevention (figures 1.2 and 1.4): primary, secondary, and tertiary prevention.

1.1.1 Primary, Secondary, and Tertiary Prevention

Type of Prevention	Intervention/Method (example)
Primary prevention	**P**revent (e.g., limit time using digital screens)
Secondary prevention	**S**creen (e.g., confrontation visual field test)
Tertiary prevention	**T**reat (e.g., cataract surgery)

Figure 1.2: Primary, secondary, and tertiary prevention.

Much of what we do in public health and healthcare is **primary prevention**. Our goal is to keep someone from getting disease or having an injury or some other health issue. Not everyone can get every health problem, but in the people that can (those that are **susceptible**) we want to create targeted messaging, use clinical markers, and work on behavioral change to reduce risks. For example, with COVID-19, our preventative messaging and actions would be to encourage vaccination, encourage mask wearing, and to stay home when sick. With ovarian cancer, however, we would not have the same discussion with every patient we might come across. If patients do not have ovaries, they are not susceptible and we do not focus on them for this particular prevention.

At some point, patients may become **exposed**, meaning that they may actually come in contact with an infectious agent or carcinogen or simply have a behavior that does something to cause pathological changes in the body. When this happens, it is not always immediately **clinically apparent**. For example, if a person is exposed to HPV, it takes time for that infection to lead to throat cancer. Until the person shows outward signs and symptoms, the disease may only be picked up via **screening**, a technique used in **secondary prevention**. Screenings help us find disease that otherwise would not be found until it reached the **clinical stage** (signs and symptoms). Patients may not be seen until the disease is clinically apparent and a stage too late for intervention, a phenomenon related to the social determinants of health. This is a reason to encourage all patients to have an annual physical exam including blood work and any additional screenings recommended by the US Preventive Services Task Force (USPSTF).[8] Our goal is to diagnose patients as often as possible when the disease is subclinical. This is called **lead time**. We'll discuss lead time and related bias in section 4.5. Screening tools do not exist for all health conditions.

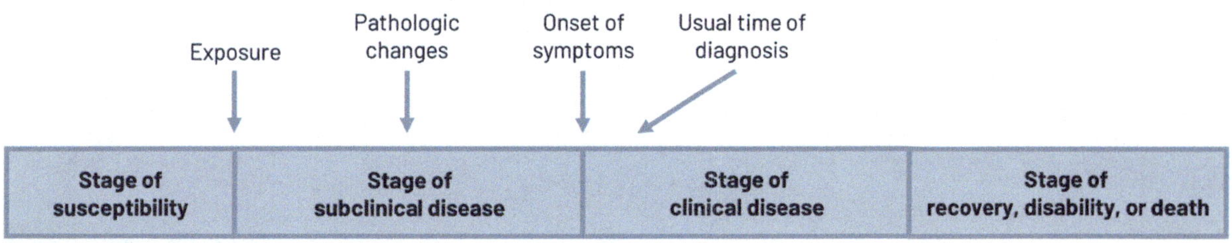

Figure 1.3: Natural history of disease timeline.

Tertiary prevention is used when the disease is already clinically apparent and we need to minimize the long-term effects of it. For example, patients with cataracts may need surgery to see better and improve their ability to perform activities of daily living. Patients with a broken femur may need surgery and rehabilitation to walk again. The ultimate goal is to prevent long-term disability and death.

Example: Physical activity as a preventative measure

For a more complete example, look at figure 1.4. If we want to prevent noncommunicable diseases (e.g., diabetes), we can use physical activity as a preventative measure. Of course, it is not the only component in preventing noncommunicable diseases but is a known tool to reduce risks. In this figure we see something called **primordial prevention** appear before primary prevention. When we think of the difference between the two, often we think about what we can do to prevent problems in our healthiest of patients. If we take a public health perspective, this would include making green space available to more of the population to encourage physical activity. From a clinical perspective, we want to encourage physical activity among all of our patients. When our patients begin to have risk factors for chronic disease, such as high blood pressure, being physically inactive, or high central adiposity (body fat), we may want to encourage higher levels of physical activity and work with patients and specialists to target their particular barriers to achieving more physical activity and exercise (primary prevention). If patients develop prediabetes, for example, we have now entered the secondary prevention area. We need to try even more tactics to improve their physical activity level and reduce their risk for development of Type II diabetes. We want to involve specialists such as nutritionists and life coaches in addition to exercise specialists to stop and reverse the course the patient is on. If none of these things work or the biologic component (e.g., family history, malabsorption of vitamins and minerals, or other conditions that preclude more activity or the benefit from activity), the patient may progress to Type II diabetes (tertiary prevention). We must continue working with this patient and specialists to minimize the long-term effects of their diabetes and encourage a long and healthy life.

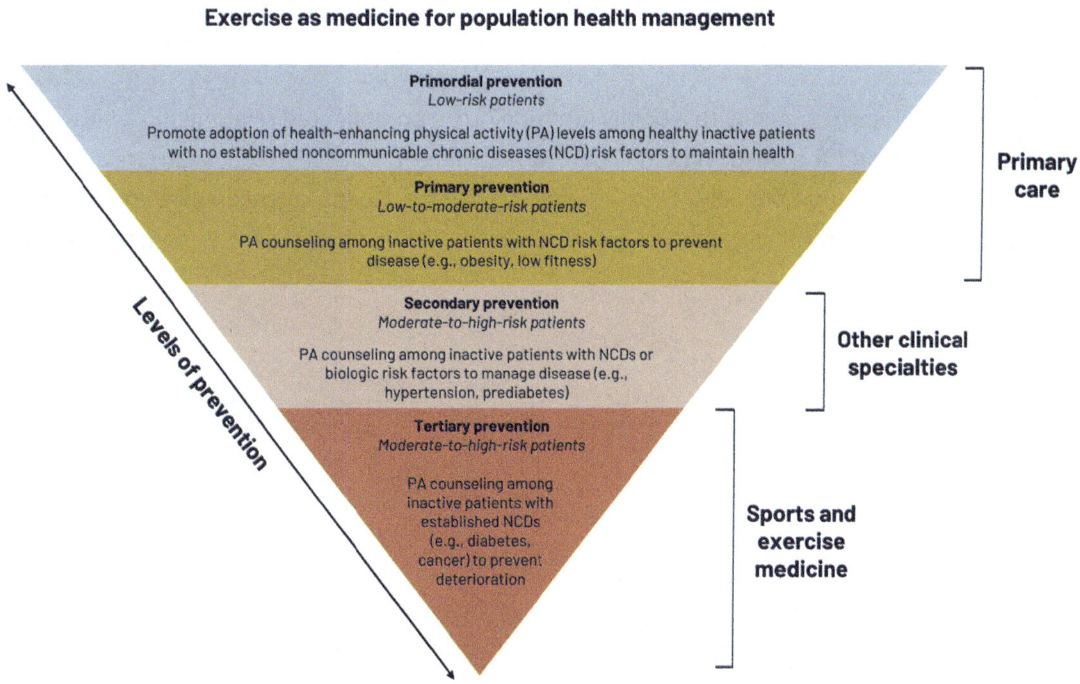

Figure 1.4: What if we want to prevent noncommunicable diseases?

As we examine topics in this book, we will use a subspecialty of *injury epidemiology*—**sports and recreation injury epidemiology (SRI)**—for examples. Other subfields of epidemiology can be found in section 1.3.

Example: Concussion in soccer

People who play soccer are considered susceptible to concussion. There are varying amounts of susceptibility—some players play every day and others play once a week. For this particular health issue, the time between exposure and the event may be long, but the time between the event and onset of symptoms is often short. It might be apparent that an athlete has a concussion, yet prior to diagnosis by a clinician there is only a presumption of a concussion. To prevent longer-term problems, the type of care a patient immediately receives as well as the care they get even after symptoms diminish are critically important.

1.2 Causality and Disease Prevention

1.2.1 Causality

Disease ("when something is wrong with a bodily function"[9]) is a complicated relationship[10] between factors of the **agent**, the **host**, and the **environment** (figure 1.5). Different diseases require different balances and interactions of these three components. Development of appropriate, practical, and effective public health measures to control or prevent disease usually requires assessment of all three components and their interactions.

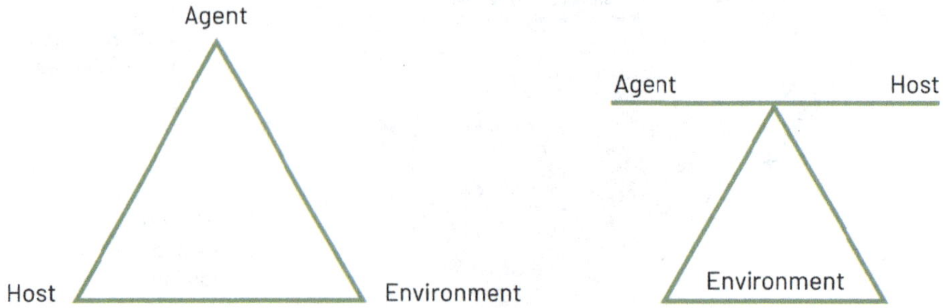

Figure 1.5: The epidemiology triangle.

An **agent** is the thing that causes disease or injury. An agent can be chemical, biological, radioactive, or environmental. Most often we think of infectious agents such as viruses. However, for many diseases, just having the presence of an agent is not **sufficient** enough to cause disease. We must also consider **pathogenicity** (ability to cause disease) and **dose** ("amount of a substance available for interaction with metabolic processes or biologically significant receptors"[11]). Some diseases, especially chronic diseases, have multiple potential causes that must be evaluated on a case-by-case basis.

The **host** is the human or creature that can get the disease. Intrinsic factors about the host influence their **exposure**, their **susceptibility** to the disease, and their **response** to whatever causes the disease or injury. Our exposures are linked to our behaviors and social determinants of health, such as our sexual practices, hygiene, diet, physical activity patterns, occupation, and personal choices. Whether or not an exposure affects us is linked to how susceptible we are and our body's response to the agent. Immunocompromised patients or patients with particular genetic features may respond differently to certain conditions, while a person's anatomic structure may make them more susceptible to other conditions. There are a number of different factors about the host that influence susceptibility, including their medications and disease.

The **environment** in the epidemiological triangle refers to the extrinsic factors about the host *and* factors that support the agent. Social determinants of health such as neighborhood flood risk, air quality, sanitation, clean water, and access to health care are signs that the environment may encourage disease or injury. Poor drainage or the presence of invasive species may encourage a poor climate that encourages insects such as mosquitoes that can transmit disease.

While epidemiology often helps prove that one thing has an influence on or directly causes another thing, the idea of **causality** (causing an effect) is complex. The **Bradford Hill Criteria**[12] (figure 1.6) are a good starting place when deciding whether a particular something (a **risk factor**, an action, etc.) is the thing or a part of things that *cause* a disease or health problem. These criteria are not requirements to prove causality, but we can consider them sometimes as strong suggestions. If we remove an actual **cause** of disease, we expect that there is then a lower risk of the occurrence of the outcome (e.g., disease or injury). There can be more than one cause of any health outcome (see below for more on multicausality). The more of these items in the Bradford Hill Criteria that are true, the more believable the possibility that the "factor" causes the outcome of interest. However, one study result does not prove causality no matter how many of the Bradford Hill Criteria are met. It takes a mountain of evidence, a solid combination of study types, and a variety of populations being examined to have strong evidence of causality.

Criteria	Description
Strength	How strong is the association between the exposure and the disease?
Consistency	Is this result repeatable by different researchers, in different populations, and at different times?
Specificity	Is the magnitude of the association stronger in one group compared to another group?
Temporality	Which comes first - the "cause" or the "effect"?
Biological gradient	Is there a dose-response relationship between the exposure and the disease?
Plausibility	Based on what we know today is this relationship at all probable?
Coherence	Does this even make sense?
Experiment	If we do an experiment, can we show the cause leads to the effect?
Analogy	Is there an established situation where a similar exposure comparably led to disease?

Figure 1.6: What are the Bradford Hill Criteria for causation?

Sometimes we simply do not know *why* answers are different between studies. We always need to acknowledge that we have varying amounts of uncertainty when examining relationships and causality. Our research to find certainty (or causality), leads us to identify factors that are **associated** with or create risk for disease or a health-event. To be a **risk factor**,

- The exposure must precede the onset of disease,
- The frequency of disease must vary by the value of the exposure, and
- The observed association must not be due to error.

We can often identify the specific action that resulted in a concussion in sports, such as heading the ball, running into a wall, falling, or getting hit. In addition to plotting our prevention on a timeline, as seen in figure 1.3, subfields of epidemiology (presented in section 1.3.2) often create and refine tools to help identify where to intervene. In SRI, Van Mechlen's Injury Prevention Sequence[13] (figure 1.7) is an example of this. In order to prevent an SRI, we must first know the *distribution* (**"Step 1: Establishing the extent of the injury problem"**). We must then know the *determinants* (**"Step 2: Establishing the etiology and mechanisms of the injury"**). We can use those two pieces of information to *apply* some intervention that can allow us to *control* SRI (**"Step 3: Introducing a preventative measure"**). After this, we need to evaluate what we did and how it worked (**"Step 4: Assessing the effectiveness"**). As seen in figure 1.7, this process is cyclical. If we succeed, the extent of the problem should be lessened. We want to eventually make the problem not a problem.

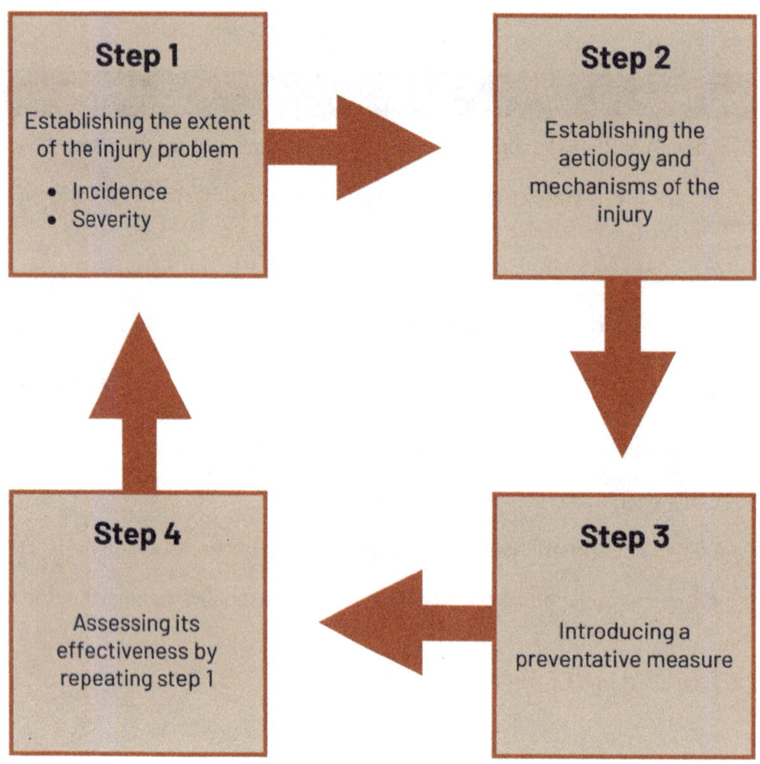

Figure 1.7: Van Mechelen's four-step "sequence of prevention."

The next figure shows how this works when applied to injuries to volleyball players.

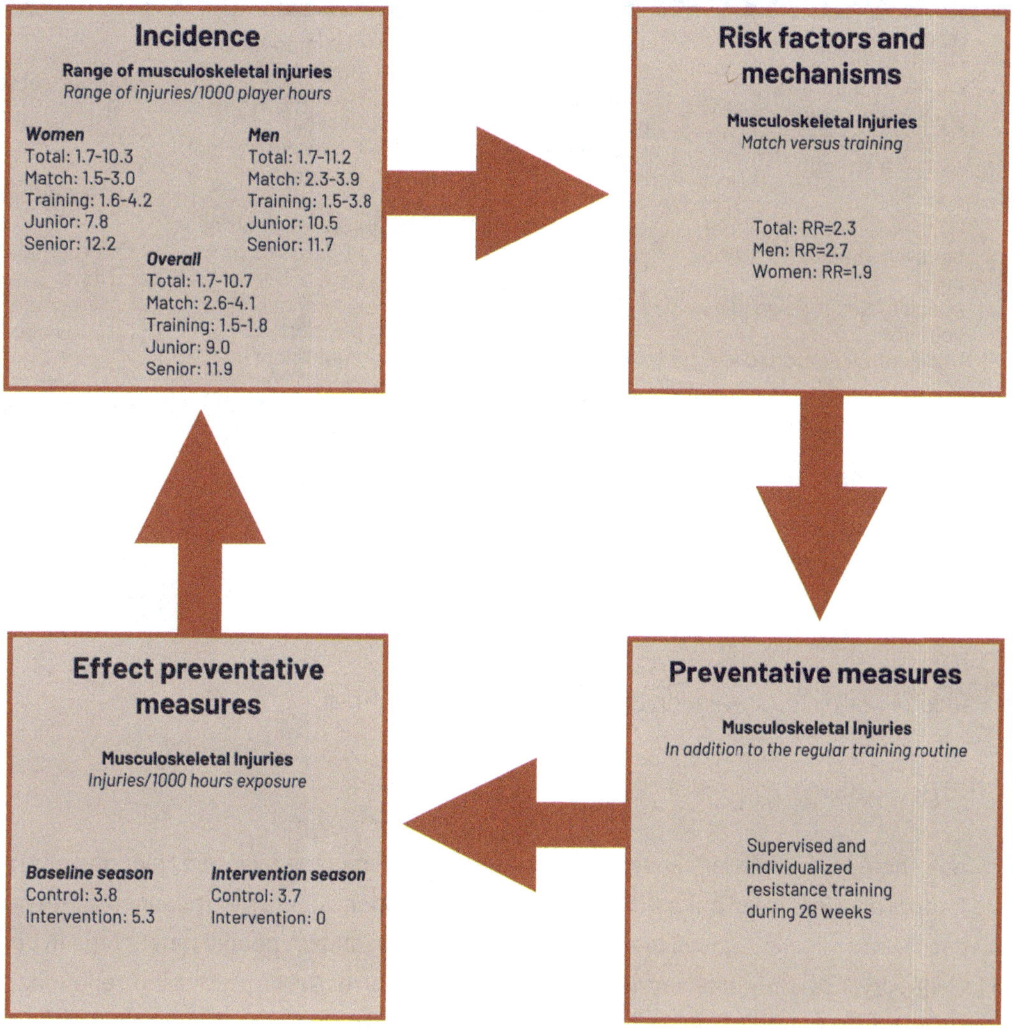

Figure 1.8: Example of the four-step "sequence of prevention" applied to injuries to volleyball players.

If we extend the idea of the four-step intervention to primary, secondary, and tertiary prevention, we might use an injury tool called Haddon's Matrix.[14] It was originally created for designing the prevention of motor vehicle crashes. Figure 1.9 presents an example for the prevention of traumatic brain injury (TBI) in baseball and softball.[15] In Haddon's Matrix, primary prevention is called "pre-injury," secondary prevention is called "injury," and tertiary prevention is called "post-injury." Measures for prevention can be applied to the host (the athlete), the agent (the thing that can hurt the athlete), the physical environment (the built environment), and the social/economic environment (nonphysical environmental factors such as **social determinants of health** [discussed later in this chapter]).

Phases	Host	Agent	Physical Environment	Social/Economic Environment
Pre-injury	• Velocity of pitch • Attitude of athlete (aggressive, competitive) • Athlete age and sex • Athlete strength	• Hardness/density of ball and bat • Inadequate protective gear • Design and type of helmet	• Maintenance of the field/grounds • Weather/time of the year • Formal/informal setting	• Public perception of wearing protective gear • Costs of protective gear
Injury	• Unaware of the potential dangers of equipment (e.g., bat) • Lack of supervision of younger athletes • Lack of education to kids	• Hardness of the ball/bat • Association of bat and ball exit velocity	• Surface hardness • Obstacles on field • Personal protective equipment	• Enforcement of rules and laws • Enforcement of protective gear use
Post-injury	• Knowledge to report symptoms • Compliance with return-to-play guidelines	• Engineering-improved helmet, bat, and ball design	• Access to a hospital or trauma center	• Expense/cost of medical system • Evaluation of surveillance systems • Insurance rates, fines • Social support • Community response to traumatic brain injury

Figure 1.9: Haddon's Matrix for prevention of TBI in baseball and softball.

1.2.2 Multicausality

No matter what, there is no singular cause of any disease. As seen in the example Haddon's Matrix in figure 1.9, multiple factors play into a TBI before it happens, when it happens, and after it happens. The same is true for other diseases, including infectious ones. Take COVID-19 for example; people must come in contact with the virus. More importantly, they must come in contact with enough of the virus for a long enough time and be susceptible to getting the virus. People who work particular jobs (e.g., ICU nurses, cashiers at convenience stores, and educators) are at higher risk, or more susceptible, to coming in contact with COVID-19 than people who telework and pick up all of their necessities using curbside pickup. This susceptibility, of course, is also tempered by each individual person's health status, vaccination status, and age, among other factors.

The factors we consider about the distribution of disease could be summed up as the overlapping factors of who is affected (**person**), where disease occurs (**place**), and when disease occurs (**time**). In **descriptive epidemiology** we quantify our population and the problem by these three factors:

- **Person** includes any and all characteristics of the patients affected by the outcome we are interested in. Examples include age, sex, gender, race, ethnicity, religion, education, behaviors, housing status, and occupation. We can use this information to better describe and examine who is affected by particular conditions, who is more likely to have particular risk factors, and overall what those affected have in common.

- **Place** makes us think not just about geographic or physical locations for those that are affected but the characteristics of those places as well. We want to know where people live, where they got sick, where they sought care, the climate of these places, the type of facilities they live or work in, the places that they eat, and anything else that could inform their susceptibility, response, or exposure to a disease. Examples include the zip code where the event occurred, whether disease occurred in a rural area, and whether or not the climate was arid.
- **Time**, as we might guess, has to do with when the outcome or exposure occurred. We want to know not just a time as in an hour of the day but a day of the week, time of the year, whether the event occurred after some other event, or if all events happened at the same time. Examples include daybreak, flu season, after a rock slide, at a potluck, or the first day of the work week.

Below is an example of how we might share this descriptive epidemiological information with others. It is a typical "Table 1," or the first table usually shown in an epidemiological or clinical paper. This table is our first look at a study population and describes each factor about them.

Example: Person and time

In a 2020 paper, Newton et al. describe the characteristics of Medicaid-insured children with sports- and nonsports-related concussion before and after Ohio's 2013 concussion law.[16]

	Pre-law		Post-law		Overall		
	n(%)		n(%)		n(%)		P-Value[b]
Total	**2742 (44.5)**		**3415 (55.5)**		**6157 (100)**		
Sex[a]							0.982
Male	1751	-64.1	2187	-64	3938	-64	
Female	982	-35.9	1228	-36	2210	-36	
Age at first visit							0.0001
5	546	-19.9	421	-12.3	967	-15.7	
5-9	484	-17.7	630	-18.5	1114	-18.1	
10-14	879	-32.1	1274	-37.3	2153	-35	
15-18	833	-30.3	1090	-31.9	1923	-31.2	
Sports-related	**726 (39.9)**		**1095 (60.1)**		**1821 (29.6)**		
Sex							0.172
Male	583	-80.3	850	-77.6	1433	-78.7	
Female	143	-19.7	245	-22.4	388	-21.3	
Age at first visit							0.012
5	24	-3.3	13	-1.2	37	-2	
5-9	97	-13.4	156	-14.2	253	-13.9	
10-14	359	-49.4	573	-52.3	932	-51.2	
15-18	246	-33.9	353	-32.2	599	-32.9	
Nonsports-related	**2016 (46.5)**		**2320 (53.5)**		**4336 (70.4)**		
Sex[a]							0.706
Male	1168	-58.2	1.337	-57.6	2505	-57.9	
Female	839	-41.8	983	-42.4	1822	-42.1	
Age at first visit							0.0001
5	522	-25.9	408	-17.6	930	-21.4	
5-9	387	-19.2	474	-20.4	861	-19.9	
10-14	520	-25.8	701	-30.2	1221	-28.2	
15-18	587	-29.1	737	-31.8	1324	-30.5	

[a]There are nine injuries with missing sex.

[b]*P*-values are based on chi-square tests of the distribution of sex and age across the law period.

Figure 1.10: Injury rates by person: Participant demographics by sports- and nonsports-related concussions, sex, and age, from pre- to post-law period, 2008-2016.

In addition to describing the population, Newton also showed the rates of concussion over time before and after the law was enacted.

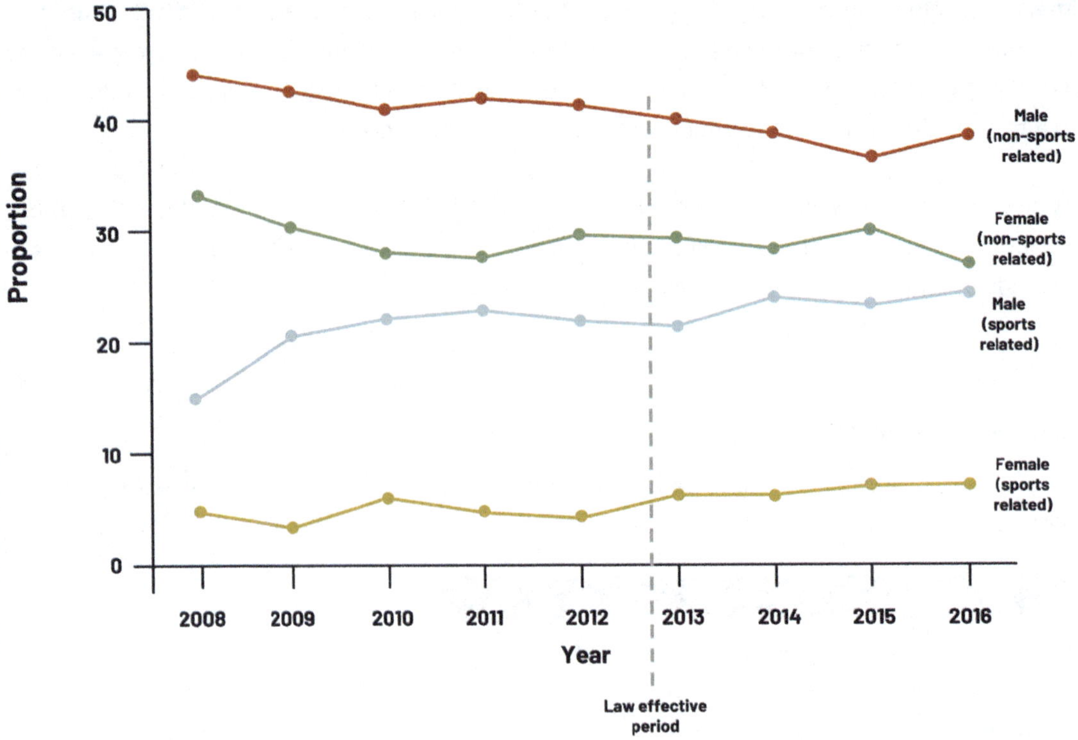

Figure 1.11: Change in the proportion of sports- and nonsports-related concussions in Medicaid-insured children by sex, from pre- to post-law period, 2008–2016.

Example: Person and place

Our next example includes data on person and place from a study of single-sport specialization during youth by present-day professional baseball players.[17] In table 1.12 we see that people can be described not just by their demographic characteristics. Players are described by their level of professional baseball and the position they play. In figure 1.13, we see a geographic display of where players lived when they first started specializing in one sport.

	n (%)
Level	
Rookie	336 (20.7)
A	578 (35.6)
AA	224 (13.8)
AAA	166 (10.2)
MLB	320 (19.7)
Total	1624
Position	
Pitcher	902 (55.4)
Starting pitcher	413
Relief pitcher	482
Infield	333 (20.4)
Outfield	249 (15.3)
Catcher	145 (8.9)
Total	1629

Figure 1.12: Level and position of all players: [a]MLB, Major League Baseball.

State	Percentage
California	19.29
Florida	12.79
Texas	12.79
Georgia	7.13
New York	3.77
North Carolina	3.56
Arizona	3.14
Illinois	2.94
New Jersey	2.73
Tennessee	2.73
Virginia	2.73
Maryland	2.31
Ohio	2.1
Washington	2.1
Alabama	1.89
Pennsylvania	1.47
South Carolina	1.47

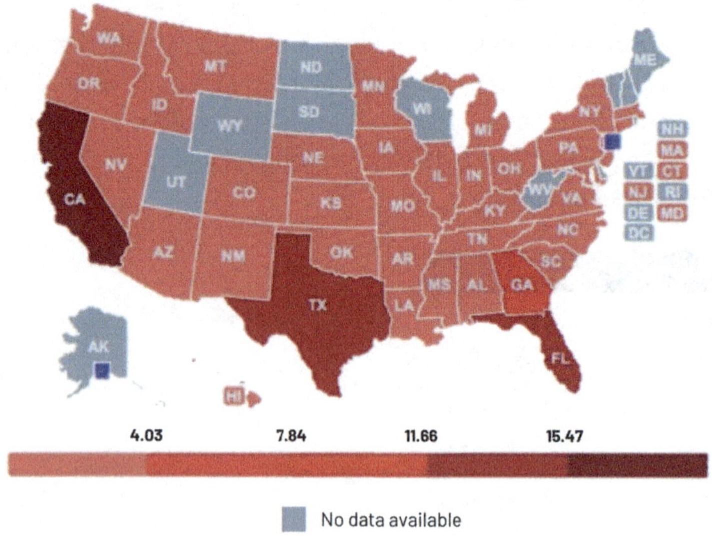

Figure 1.13: MLB player state of residence when beginning to specialize in baseball.

Once we start looking at the problem by person, place, and time, we also have to identify our best estimate as to how the particular case or cases of disease occurred. **Rothman's Pie Model**[18] (figure 1.14) is an example of how we can consider the multicausality of disease or health-related events.

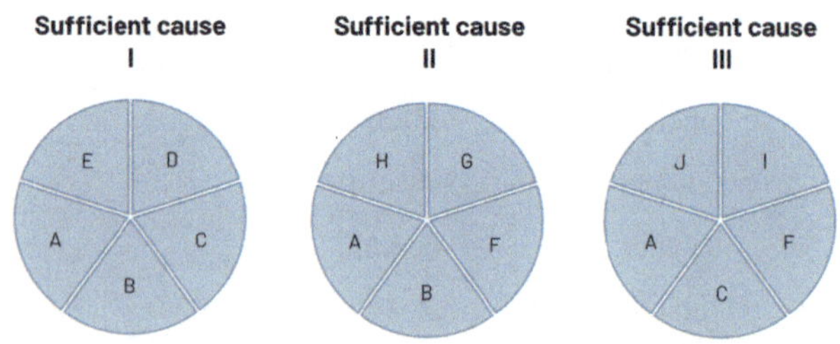

Figure 1.14: Rothman's Pie Model (Disclaimer: Each pie in figure 1.14 has five pieces, but that in no way means that every disease has five factors that cause it; this is just an example).

- Each completed pie (**sufficient cause**) is a case (person) of a single disease. Figure 1.14 demonstrates that the same disease may have more than one sufficient cause. Consider that two people with a TBI do not have to have the same factors that contributed to their TBI or recovery from it (sufficient cause I, II, III).
- Each individual pie piece (or **component cause**) is the equivalent of an individual factor that contributes to causing disease (A, B, C, D, E, F, G, H, I, J).
- If a piece of the pie is present in every pie, it is considered a **necessary cause**. In figure 1.14, piece A is in every pie. We do not know whether every disease or health-related event has a necessary cause. Some, such as COVID-19, do. If a person has every factor in common with a person who has COVID-19 but did not come in contact with the virus, that person will not have COVID-19.

Component causes can be proximal (downstream), medial (midstream), and distal (upstream) to the health-related event (figure 1.14). In both clinical and public health matters it can often be very important to know which particular risk factors or component causes are present. For example, focusing on a patient's lack of physical activity (risk factor for disease) when they come in for an annual visit without knowing more details about why they are not getting enough physical activity likely will not change the patient's behavior. However, if you know that the patient works three jobs to feed the family (proximal), you may be able to find small ways to help them increase their activity level. Continue asking why and you'll eventually get to the distal causes. These component causes are where we should focus our primordial and primary prevention efforts.

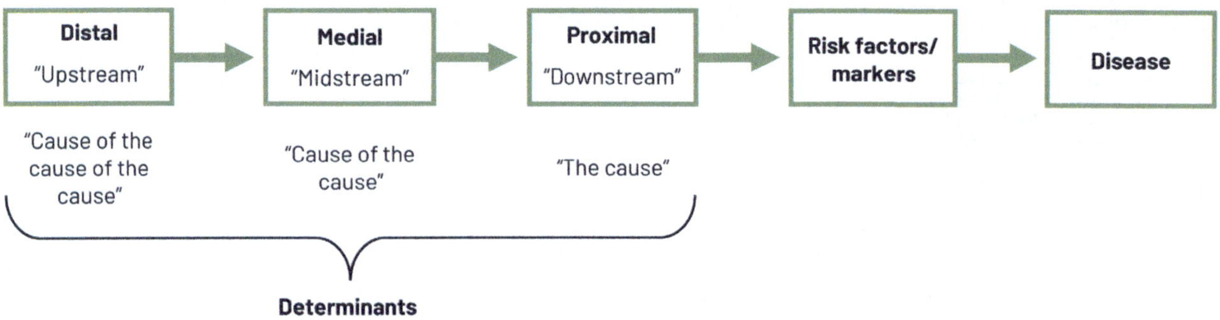

Figure 1.15: Examples of social determinants of health.

What are some more examples? Figure 1.16 shows an example of how component causes contribute to sports injury. Factors about a person such as age, physical fitness, and anatomy (**internal risk factors**) make an athlete predisposed to injury. Being exposed to external risk factors, such as particular equipment or a hazardous playing environment, influences the predisposed athlete and results in one now susceptible to injury. Finally, something (**an inciting event**) must occur, such as the player planting a foot on the turf in a particular way to cause an injury.

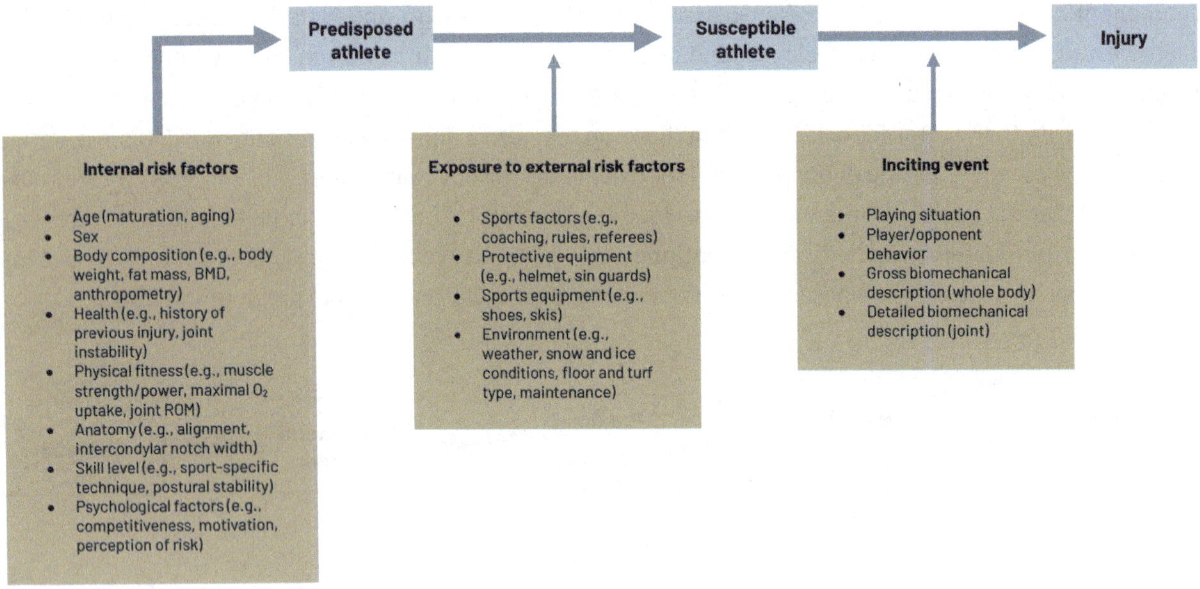

Figure 1.16: Comprehensive model for injury causation.

Social determinants of health (SDOH)[19] (figure 1.17) are the conditions in the environments where people are born, live, learn, work, play, worship, and age that affect a wide range of health, functioning, and quality-of-life outcomes and risks. Social determinants are issues that affect the people we study; what we ask or measure in our studies; what we consider as solutions; or whose diseases matter the most. Each of these factors holds its own importance in health.

Economic stability	Neighborhood and physical environment	Education	Food	Community and social context	Health care system
• Employment • Income • Expenses • Debt • Medical bills • Support	• Housing • Transportation • Safety • Parks • Playgrounds • Walkability • Zip code/ geography	• Literacy • Language • Early childhood education • Vocational training • Higher education	• Hunger • Access to healthy options	• Social integration • Support systems • Community engagement • Discrimination • Stress	• Health coverage • Provider availability • Provider linguistic and cultural competency • Quality of care
Health outcomes: mortality, morbidity, life expectancy, health care expenditures, health status, functional limitations					

Figure 1.17: Examples of social determinants of health.

By including SDOH in epidemiological work, we can make progress toward achieving **health equity** (figure 1.18). These factors are all quite important when we consider a person or community's risk for disease, the probability they have for getting adequate care, and the probability for achieving health professionals' intended outcome from prevention efforts.

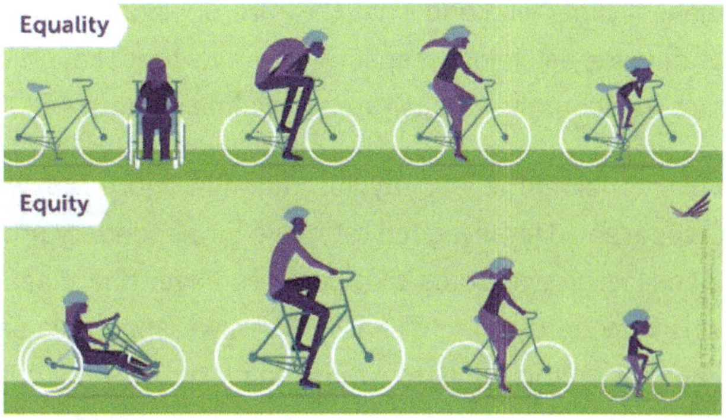

Figure 1.18: Health equality versus equity.

In order to achieve **health equity, health disparities must be addressed.** Health disparities are not simple differences in health status. They are differences in health outcomes between populations that are tied to race, ethnicity, sex, gender, age, disability, SES, and geography. By describing the health of the population, we can identify what health disparities exist so we can do something about them.

1.2.3 Clinically Apparent Disease

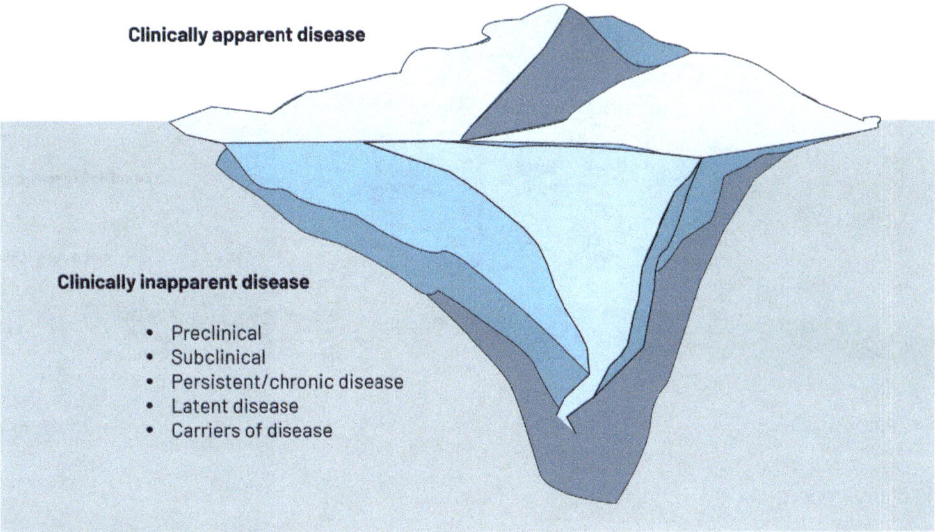

Figure 1.19: Clinically apparent versus clinically inapparent disease.

When we consider the universe of disease or health-related states, we must also recognize that some existing diseases are not immediately apparent. This contributes to fluctuation in our understanding of disease and disease patterns. It also contributes to changes in our observed burden of disease or how we decide what resources are needed for our community. For example, a large percentage of people with SRI do not seek care in a clinical system. Many of our estimates of the prevalence of SRI, however, are based on how many appear in an emergency department or other clinical centers. Epidemiologists have a responsibility to make it clear who and what they are considering when discussing disease. Figures 1.19 and 1.20, icebergs of disease and injury respectively, show that though we might see some aspects of disease or injury, most factors about the disease are not visible without looking below the surface.

If we consider the iceberg illustration in figure 1.19, we see that much of the disease that exists is clinically inapparent. This is a good rationale for secondary prevention. We need ways to find and address persistent diseases or symptoms that patients have, find disease that is not yet causing symptoms, and find those who may be carrying disease. When we apply this same concept to the causes of injury (figure 1.20), we see that factors we notice most about disease are ones we can easily "diagnose"—things that are biological, things that are psychological, and things that are caused by behaviors of patients.[20] However, most injury is driven by a host of other factors, including relationships with family and friends (**interpersonal**), where people work and play (**organizational**), societal norms and community resources (**community**), and policies (**society**). Different people have different risks.

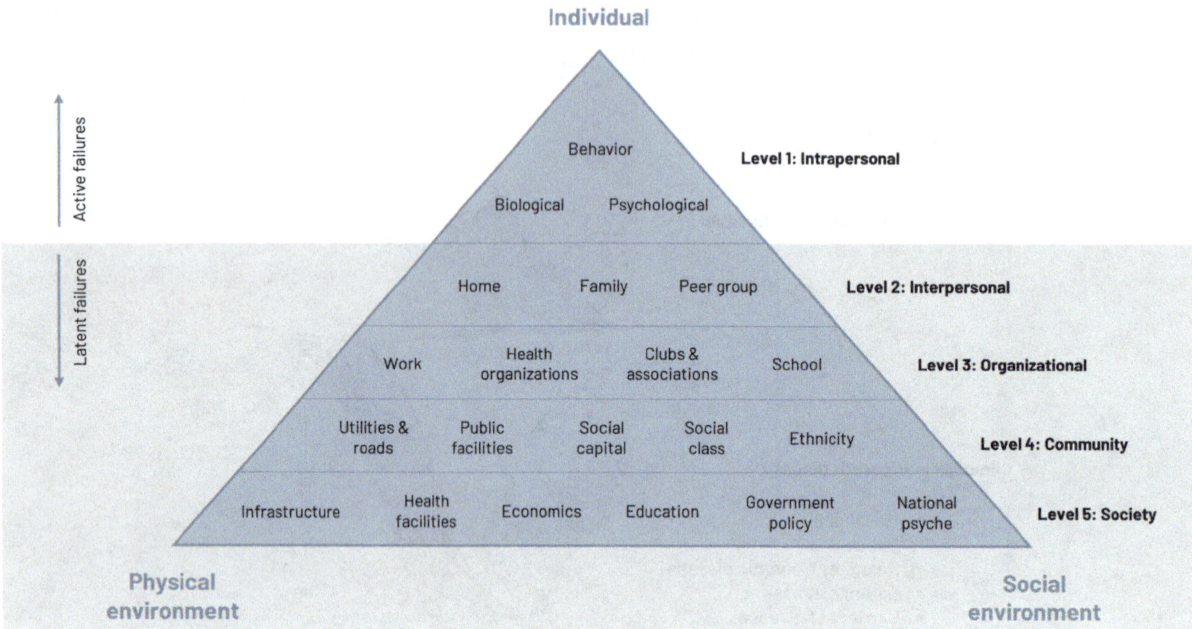

Figure 1.20: The injury iceberg.

Further reading

Check out this real-life example of how we can examine the COVID-19 pandemic in the US by county in real time.[21]

1.3 The Importance of Epidemiology in Your Research

As seen throughout the first part of this chapter, epidemiology is a broad subject that studies the distribution and determinants of health-related states or events (including disease).[22,23] This section and the rest of the text focus on the application of this study to the control of diseases and other health problems.[24,25] Specifically, there are two major uses of epidemiology: (1) describing the status of the population's health and the health services of the population and (2) determining or describing the etiology of diseases, conditions, syndromes, and so on. Nearly everything epidemiology is used for in public health and clinical medicine falls within these two uses. We also recognize that when we think about epidemiology, we can consider that we use it to describe the *who, what, where, when, why*, and *how* of disease. All of these factors are important for research and for helping patients every day. We conclude this section with a list of some of the subspecialty areas of epidemiology. Each of these areas has very specific methods that are important to helping people and each of them may have a more direct impact on the work you do in clinical settings than others. You do not need to remember each of these areas, but do know that you can find subject-matter experts for nearly any problem you face!

1.3.1 Uses of Epidemiology

There are two major uses of epidemiology:

1. Describing the status of the population's health and the health services of the population
    - Health services research
        - How do our services work?
        - Are the services in the right place?
        - Is utilization adequate? Who is not using the services?
        - Appropriateness of staffing and facilities
        - Diagnose the health of the community
        - History of the health of populations
    - Policy
        - Create or evaluate the policies that affect health
    - Health promotion/health behavior
    - Social science
    - History
        - Where have we been?
        - Where are we going?
        - Look at long-term trend
            1. What causes changes in our numbers?
            2. Were there changes in our diagnosis, etiology, or reporting criteria?
        - Identify at-risk populations

- Note improvements or declines in health

2. Determining or describing the etiology of diseases, conditions, syndromes, etc.
    - Biology
    - Ecology
    - History
    - Laboratory sciences
    - Genetics

If epidemiology is about the *who, what, where, when, why*, and *how* of disease:

Descriptive epidemiology is about *who, what, where*, and *when.*

Analytic epidemiology is about *why* and *how.*

1.3.2 Subfields of Epidemiology

In addition to injury epidemiology, subareas or subfields of epidemiology include:

- infectious disease epidemiology
- chronic disease epidemiology
- pharmacoepidemiology
- legal epidemiology
- cardiovascular epidemiology
- cancer epidemiology
- oral health epidemiology
- methods epidemiology
- clinical epidemiology
- aging epidemiology
- genetic epidemiology
- neuro epidemiology
- psychiatric epidemiology
- nutritional epidemiology
- reproductive epidemiology
- perinatal epidemiology
- pediatric epidemiology
- applied public health epidemiology
- global health epidemiology
- diabetes epidemiology
- clinical trials epidemiology
- molecular epidemiology
- physical activity epidemiology
- women's health epidemiology
- men's health epidemiology
- social epidemiology
- environmental epidemiology
- field epidemiology
- veterinary epidemiology

While this is not an exhaustive list of subareas of epidemiology, they do represent much of the expertise available. Because of the breadth of subspecialties, when searching for literature on any given topic you are likely to find at least some epidemiological papers available. Peer-reviewed epidemiology manuscripts are in a large variety of journals, including many that do not use the word "epidemiology" in the title. Many epidemiology papers can be found using academic library resources (such as those from the University Libraries at Virginia Tech[26]), PubMed,[27] or Google Scholar.[28]

Figure Descriptions

Figure 1.1: Boxed chart with x- and y- axis. On x-axis is age groups, on y-axis is rank. Example causes include suicide, heart disease, COVID-19, etc. The main group highlighted in this table is unintentional injury. Distribution of unintentional injury is ranked fourth for age group <1 and 55-64, first for age groups 1-44, third for age group 45-54, and eighth for age group 65+. Return to figure 1.1.

Figure 1.3: Timeline from left to right: stage of susceptibility, exposure, stage of subclinical disease (pathologic changes occur here), onset of symptoms, stage of clinical disease (time of diagnosis usually occurs at the beginning of this stage), and stage of recovery, disability, or death. Return to figure 1.3.

Figure 1.4: Exercise as medicine for population health management represented as an upside down triangle with 4 levels of prevention. Top 2 levels of prevention: primary care, middle level: other clinical specialties, bottom level: sports and exercise medicine. Top level: Primordial prevention (low risk patients). Promote adoption of health-enhancing physical activity (PA) levels among healthy inactive patients with no established non communicable chronic diseases (NCD) risk factors to maintain health. Next level: Primary prevention (low-to-moderate risk patients). PA counseling among inactive patients with NCD risk factors to prevent disease (e.g., obesity, low fitness). Next level: Secondary prevention (moderate-to-high risk patients). PA counseling among inactive patients with NCDs or biologic risk factors to manage disease (e.g., hypertension, pre-diabetes). Bottom level: Tertiary prevention (moderate-to-high risk patients). PA counseling among inactive patients with established NCDs (e.g., diabetes, cancer) to prevent deterioration. Return to figure 1.4.

Figure 1.5: One triangle model shows agent, host, and environment in three corners as having equal influence. Another model shows agent and host as interdependent variables (like a balance beam), with the environment at the base of the triangle. The environment has influence on the balance of agent and host. Return to figure 1.5.

Figure 1.7: Step 1: establishing the extent of the injury problem (incidence, severity). Step 2: establishing the etiology and mechanisms of the injury. Step 3: introducing a preventative measure. Step 4: Assessing its effectiveness by repeating step 1. Return to figure 1.7.

Figure 1.8: Step 1: Incidence (range of musculoskeletal injuries measured in injuries per 1000 player hours). Women (total: 1.7-10.3, match: 1.5-3.0, training: 1.6-4.2, junior: 7.8, senior: 12.2). Men (total: 1.7-11.2, match: 2.3-3.9, training: 1.5-3.8, junior: 10.5, senior: 11.7). Overall (total: 1.7-10.7, match: 2.6-4.1, training: 1.5-1.8, junior: 9, senior: 11.9). Step 2: risk factors and mechanisms (musculoskeletal injuries in matches versus training). Total: RR=2.3, Men: RR=2.7, Women: RR=1.9. Step 3: Preventive measures (musculoskeletal injuries in addition to the regular training routine). Supervised and individualized resistance training during 26 weeks. Step 4: effect preventive measures (musculoskeletal injuries measured in injuries per 1000 hours of exposure). Baseline season (control: 3.8, intervention: 5.3). Intervention season (control: 3.7, intervention: 0). Arrow goes back to step 1. Return to figure 1.8.

Figure 1.11: Line graph with x- and y-axis. On x-axis is the year from 2008-2016, on y-axis is the proportion from 0-50. Law effective period is shown as a dotted vertical line between years 2012 and 2013. Following this period, the chart shows a relative decrease in non-sports-related injury for both males and females, as compared to the pre-law period. The chart also shows a relative increase for sports related concussions for males and females. Return to figure 1.11.

Figure 1.13: Heat map of USA shows states with the highest percentage of MLB player state of residence. From highest to lowest. California: 19.29, Florida: 12.79, Texas: 12.79, Georgia: 7.13, New York: 3.77, North Carolina: 3.56, Arizona: 3.14, Illinois: 2.94, New Jersey: 2.73, Tennessee: 2,73, Virginia: 2.73, Maryland: 2.31, Ohio: 2.1, Washington: 2.1, Alabama: 1,89, Pennsylvania: 1.47, South Carolina: 1.47. Return to figure 1.13.

Figure 1.14: Causal pies are pie charts with each component cause as a slice. Three pies with sufficient causes I, II, III. Slice A is in each pie. Slice B is only in pies 1 and 2. Slice C is only in pies 1 and 3. Return to figure 1.14.

Figure 1.15: From left to right. Distal (upstream or the cause of the cause of the cause), Medial (midstream or the cause of the cause), Proximal (downstream or the cause), risk factors/markers, disease. Distal, medial, and proximal are determinants. Return to figure 1.15.

Figure 1.16: From left to right. Internal risk factors, predisposed athlete, exposure to external risk factors, susceptible athlete, inciting event, injury. Internal risk factors: age (maturation, aging), sex, body composition (e.g., body weight, fat mass, BMD, anthropometry), health (e.g., history of previous injury, joint instability), physical fitness (e.g., muscle strength/power, maximal O2 uptake, joint ROM), anatomy (e.g., alignment, intercondylar notch width), skill level (e.g., sport scientific technique, postural stability), psychological factors (e.g., competitiveness, motivation, perception of risk). Exposure to external risk factors: sports factors (e.g., coaching, rules, referees), protective equipment (e.g., helmet, shin guards), sports equipment (e.g., shoes, skis), environment (e.g., weather, snow and ice conditions, floor and turf type, maintenance). Inciting event: playing situation, player/opponent behavior, gross biomechanical description (whole body), detailed biomechanical description (joint). Return to figure 1.16.

Figure 1.18: Equality: giving everyone the same bike. Equity: giving everyone a bike that works for them (i.e., adapted bike for wheelchair users, smaller bikes for smaller people, etc.). Return to figure 1.18.

Figure 1.19: Visible part of the iceberg: clinically apparent disease. Hidden part of the iceberg (under water): clinically inapparent disease (preclinical, subclinical, persistent/chronic disease, latent disease, carriers of disease). Return to figure 1.19.

Figure 1.20: Triangle with 5 horizontal sections connecting triangle's 3 corners: individual (top), physical environment (bottom left), and social environment (bottom right). First horizontal section is Level 1 (intrapersonal): behavior, biological, psychological. These are active failures, and are often more clinically apparent and diagnosable. Level 2 (interpersonal): home, family, peer group. Level 3 (organizational): work, health organizations, clubs and associations, school. Level 4 (community): utilities and roads, public facilities, social capital, social class, ethnicity. Level 5 (society): infrastructure, health facilities, economics, education, government policy, national psyche. Levels 2-5 are latent failures and represent inapparent disease, or the hidden part of the iceberg. Return to figure 1.20.

Figure References

Figure 1.1: Ten leading causes of death in the United States, 2020. Kindred Grey. 2022. CC BY 4.0. Data from https://wisqars.cdc.gov/fatal-leading.

Figure 1.2: Primary, secondary, and tertiary prevention. Adapted under fair use from USMLE First Aid, Step 1.

Figure 1.3: Natural history of disease timeline. Kindred Grey. 2022. CC BY 4.0. Adapted from https://www.cdc.gov/csels/dsepd/ss1978/Lesson1/Section9.html#ALT118

Figure 1.4: What if we want to prevent noncommunicable diseases?. Kindred Grey. 2023. Adapted with permission from Lobelo F, Beyond citius, altius, fortius. Aspetar Sports Medicine Journal. CC BY NC SA 4.0.

Figure 1.5: The epidemiology triangle. Kindred Grey. 2022. Adapted from figure 1.16 from CDC (public domain).

Figure 1.6: What are the Bradford Hill Criteria for causation? Adapted from Hill AB. The environment and disease: Association or causation? Proc R Soc Med. 1965;58(5):295-300. DOI:10.1177/003591576505800503

Figure 1.7: Van Mechelen's four-step "sequence of prevention." Kindred Grey. 2022. Adapted under fair use from van Mechelen W, Hlobil H, Kemper HC. Incidence, severity, aetiology and prevention of sports injuries: A review of concepts. Sports Med. 1992;14:82-99. DOI: 10.2165/00007256-199214020-00002

Figure 1.8: Example of the four-step "sequence of prevention" applied to injuries to volleyball players. Kindred Grey. 2022. Adapted under fair use from Kilic O, Maas M, Verhagen E, Zwerver J, and Gouttebarge V.(2017) Incidence, aetiology and prevention of musculoskeletal injuries in volleyball: A systematic review of the literature, European Journal of Sport Science. 2017;17:6, 765-793, DOI: 10.1080/17461391.2017.1306114 (CC BY-NC-ND 4.0)

Figure 1.9: Haddon's Matrix for prevention of TBI in baseball and softball. Adapted from table 7 in Cusimano

MD and Zhu A. Systematic review of traumatic brain injuries in baseball and softball: A framework for prevention. Front. Neurol. 2017;8:492. DOI: 10.3389/fneur.2017.00492 (CC BY)

Figure 1.10: Injury rates by person. Data from Newton A, Yang J, Shi J, et al. Sports and non-sports-related concussions among Medicaid-insured children: Health care utilization before and after Ohio's concussion law. Inj Epidemiol. 2020;7(1):55. DOI:10.1186/s40621-020-00283-w (CC BY 4.0)

Figure 1.11: Change in the proportion of sports- and nonsports-related concussions in Medicaid-insured children by sex, from pre- to post-law period, 2008–2016. Kindred Grey. 2022. CC BY 4.0. Data from Newton A, Yang J, Shi J, et al. Sports and non-sports-related concussions among Medicaid-insured children: Health care utilization before and after Ohio's concussion law. Inj Epidemiol. 2020;7(1):55. DOI:10.1186/s40621-020-00283-w (CC BY 4.0)

Figure 1.12: Level and position of all players. aMLB, Major League Baseball. Data from Buckley PS, Ciccotti MC, Bishop M, et al. Youth Single-Sport Specialization in Professional Baseball Players. Orthop J Sports Med. 2020;8(3):2325967120907875. Published 2020 Mar 20. DOI:10.1177/2325967120907875 (CC BY-NC-ND)

Figure 1.13: MLB Player state of residence when beginning to specialize in baseball. Used under fair use from Buckley PS, Ciccotti MC, Bishop M, et al. Youth Single-Sport Specialization in Professional Baseball Players. Orthop J Sports Med. 2020;8(3):2325967120907875. Published 2020 Mar 20. DOI:10.1177/2325967120907875 (CC BY-NC-ND)

Figure 1.14: Rothman's pie model. Kindred Grey. 2022. Adapted under fair use from Rothman KJ. Causes. 1976. Am J Epidemiol. 1995;141(2):90-89. DOI:10.1093/oxfordjournals.aje.a117417

Figure 1.15: Examples of social determinants of health. Kindred Grey. 2022. CC BY 4.0. Adapted from Garry Egger, John Dixon, "Beyond Obesity and Lifestyle: A Review of 21st Century Chronic Disease Determinants", BioMed Research International, vol. 2014, Article ID 731685, 12 pages, 2014. DOI:10.1155/2014/731685 (CC BY 4.0)

Figure 1.16: Comprehensive model for injury causation. Kindred Grey. 2022. Adapted under fair use from Bahr R, Krosshaug TUnderstanding injury mechanisms: a key component of preventing injuries in sportBritish Journal of Sports Medicine 2005;39:324-329. DOI: 10.1136/bjsm.2005.018341

Figure 1.17: Examples of social determinants of health. Used under fair use from Social Determinants of Health - What are Payers Doing? from HealthEdge and Beyond Health Care: The Role of Social Determinants in Promoting Health and Health Equity from KFF.

Figure 1.18: Health equity versus health equality. Visualizing Health Equity: One Size Does Not Fit All Infographic by Robert Wood Johnson Foundation. 2017. CC BY-NC-ND.

Figure 1.19: Clinically apparent versus clinically inapparent disease. Kindred Grey. 2022. CC BY-SA 4.0. Includes Iceberg in the Arctic with its underside exposed001 by Pk0001 from WikimediaCommons (CC BY-SA 4.0).

Figure 1.20: The injury iceberg. Kindred Grey. 2022. Adapted under fair use from Hanson D, Hanson J, Vardon P, McFarlane K, Lloyd J, Muller R, Durrheim D. The injury iceberg: an ecological approach to planning sustainable community safety interventions. Health Promot J Austr. 2005 Apr;16(1):5-10. DOI: 10.1071/he05005

Notes

1. Bonita R, Beaglehole R, Kjellström T. *Basic Epidemiology*. World Health Organization; 2006. https://apps.who.int/iris/bitstream/handle/10665/43541/9241547073_eng.pdf. Accessed September 9, 2023.
2. Frérot M, Lefebvre A, Aho S, Callier P, Astruc K, Aho Glélé LS. What is epidemiology? Changing definitions of epidemiology 1978-2017. PloS one. 2018;13(12):e0208442.
3. Bonita R, Beaglehole R, Kjellström T. *Basic Epidemiology*. World Health Organization; 2006. https://apps.who.int/iris/

bitstream/handle/10665/43541/9241547073_eng.pdf. Accessed September 9, 2023.

4. Frérot M, Lefebvre A, Aho S, Callier P, Astruc K, Aho Glélé LS. What is epidemiology? Changing definitions of epidemiology 1978-2017. PloS one. 2018;13(12):e0208442.
5. National Center for Injury Prevention and Control, Centers for Disease Control and Prevention. 10 Leading Causes of Death, United States: 2020, All Races, Both Sexes. Web-based Injury Statistics Query and Reporting System (WISQARS)[Online]. https://wisqars.cdc.gov/data/lcd/home. Accessed September 9, 2023.
6. National Center for Health Statistics, Centers for Disease Control and Prevention. National Center for Health Statistics. https://www.cdc.gov/nchs/index.htm. Published 2022. Accessed 2022.
7. Centers for Disease Control and Prevention. Centers for Disease Control and Prevention. https://www.cdc.gov/nchs/index.htm. Published 2022. Accessed 2022.
8. U.S. Preventive Services Task Force. Recommendation Topics. https://www.uspreventiveservicestaskforce.org/uspstf/recommendation-topics. Published 2022. Accessed 2022.
9. Porta M. *A Dictionary of Epidemiology*. 6th ed. Oxford University Press; 2014.
10. U.S. Department of Health and Human Services, Centers for Disease Control and Prevention. Chain of infection. In: *Principles of Epidemiology*. 3rd ed; 2006: 1-62-1-71.
11. Porta M. *A Dictionary of Epidemiology*. 6th ed. Oxford University Press; 2014.
12. Hill AB. The environment and disease: Association or causation? Proc R Soc Med. 1965;58(5):295-300.
13. van Mechelen W, Hlobil H, Kemper HC. Incidence, severity, aetiology and prevention of sports injuries: A review of concepts. Sports medicine (Auckland, NZ). 1992;14(2):82-99.
14. Haddon W, Jr. The changing approach to the epidemiology, prevention, and amelioration of trauma: The transition to approaches etiologically rather than descriptively based. Am J Public Health Nations Health. 1968;58(8):1431-1438.
15. Cusimano MD, Zhu A. Systematic review of traumatic brain injuries in baseball and softball: A framework for prevention. Frontiers in Neurology. 2017;8(492).
16. Newton A, Yang J, Shi J, et al. Sports and non-sports-related concussions among Medicaid-insured children: Health care utilization before and after Ohio's concussion law. Inj Epidemiol. 2020;7(1):55.
17. Buckley PS, Ciccotti MC, Bishop M, et al. Youth single-sport specialization in professional baseball players. Orthop J Sports Med. 2020;8(3):2325967120907875.
18. Rothman KJ. Causes. Am J Epidemiol. 1976;104(6):587-592.
19. U.S. Department of Health and Human Services, Office of Disease Prevention and Health Promotion, Healthy People 2030. Social determinants of health. https://health.gov/healthypeople/objectives-and-data/social-determinants-health. Published 2020. Accessed October 18, 2020.
20. Hanson D, Hanson J, Vardon P, et al. The injury iceberg: An ecological approach to planning sustainable community safety interventions. Health Promotion Journal of Australia. 2005;16(1):5-10.
21. Centers for Disease Control and Prevention. COVID-19 vaccinations by county. https://covid.cdc.gov/covid-data-tracker/#county-view?list_select_state=all_states&data-type=CommunityLevels. Published 2023. Accessed September 9, 2023.
22. Bonita R, Beaglehole R, Kjellström T. *Basic Epidemiology*. World Health Organization; 2006. https://apps.who.int/iris/bitstream/handle/10665/43541/9241547073_eng.pdf. Accessed September 9, 2023.
23. Frérot M, Lefebvre A, Aho S, Callier P, Astruc K, Aho Glélé LS. What is epidemiology? Changing definitions of epidemiology 1978-2017. PloS one. 2018;13(12):e0208442.
24. Bonita R, Beaglehole R, Kjellström T. *Basic Epidemiology*. World Health Organization; 2006. https://apps.who.int/iris/bitstream/handle/10665/43541/9241547073_eng.pdf. Accessed September 9, 2023.
25. Frérot M, Lefebvre A, Aho S, Callier P, Astruc K, Aho Glélé LS. What is epidemiology? Changing definitions of epidemiology 1978-2017. PloS one. 2018;13(12):e0208442.
26. Virginia Tech. University Libraries. https://lib.vt.edu/. Published 2022. Accessed 2022.
27. PubMed [Internet]. National Library of Medicine (US). https://www.ncbi.nlm.nih.gov/pubmed/. Published 1946-2022. Accessed 2022.

28. Google Scholar. Google. https://scholar.google.com/. Published 2022. Accessed 2022.

2. MEASURING THINGS IN EPIDEMIOLOGY

2.1 Types of Counting

Epidemiologists are interested in the numbers behind health issues, including:

- How many people/animals are affected?
- How long are people/animals affected?
- Do the numbers differ by other factors?
- How many deaths are there?

Being able to do the work of an epidemiologist all comes down to *appropriately counting what happens.* There are two general categories of counting that we use in epidemiology: **counts** and **ratios. Counts** are the simplest and most frequently performed quantitative measures in epidemiology. Counts refer to the number of cases of a disease or other health phenomenon being studied. Most of the numbers you frequently see in epidemiology are types of ratios (**rates**, **proportions**, and **percentages**). **Ratios** are the values obtained by dividing one quantity (count) by another (numerator over a denominator).

Example: Interpreting ratios

Between 1981 and 2007, 2,920,260 men died of injury (any type) and 1,119,669 women died of injury (any type) in the United States (figure 2.1).[1]

Count	
Injury Deaths in Men	2,920,260
Injury Deaths in Women	1,119,669
Ratio	
2,920,260 / 1,119,669 = 2.6:1 men to women	

Figure 2.1: Injury deaths in men and women in the United States.

We would interpret this **sex ratio** by saying "Between 1981 and 2007, for every 2.6 injury deaths among men, there was one injury death among women in the United States."

We can use ratios to contrast different levels of injury severity from the most severe (e.g., death) to least severe (e.g., injured but not needing treatment) (figure 2.2). As the size and breadth of the population affected grows, the strength of definitive evidence for the marker decreases. We must strike a balance between the two when optimizing the use of the ratio.

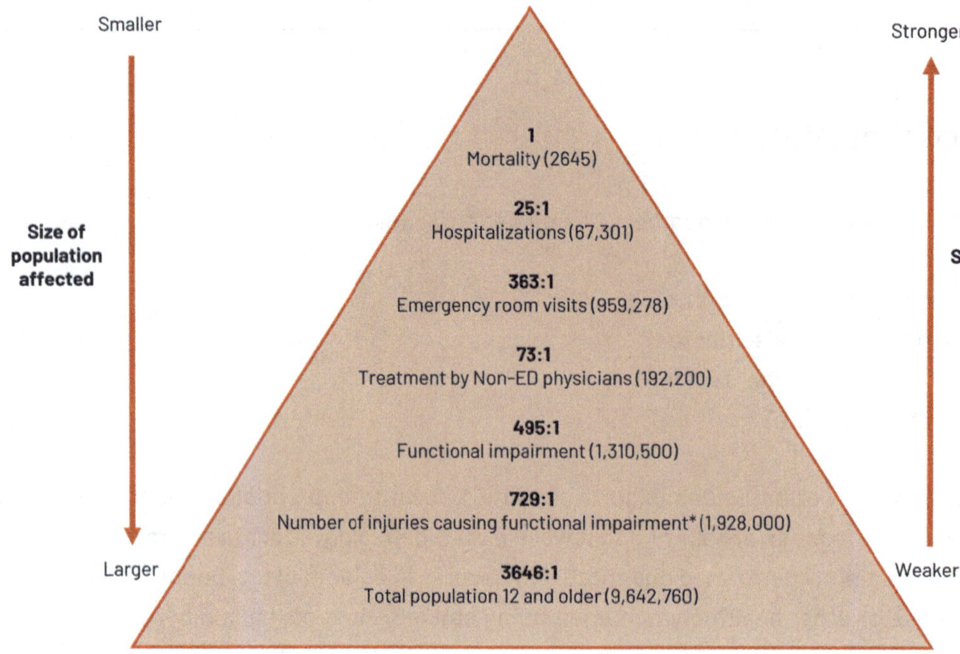

Figure 2.2: Deaths to injury severity ratio example. (*Includes multiple injuries per individual).

2.1.1 Proportions

Proportions are a measure that states a **count** *relative to* the size of the group. It is a **ratio** in which *the denominator contains the numerator*. It can be expressed (written, said, etc.) as a **percentage**. A proportion can be used to demonstrate the **magnitude** of a health problem.

Example: Magnitude

If 10 dormitory students develop strep throat, we want to know how important the problem is.

- If only 20 students live in the dorm, 50 percent are ill. *Magnitude: This is a major problem! We need action immediately.*
- If 500 students live in the dorm, 2 percent are ill. *Magnitude: This is a problem but not as concerning. We will likely keep a cautious eye on the situation but not act immediately.*

Prevalence is the number of existing cases of a disease or health condition in a population at some designated time. Prevalence is a proportion. It can be expressed (written, said, etc.,) as follows:

- A number
- A percentage
- The number of cases per unit size of the population

If no time is specified, we usually are discussing **point prevalence** or prevalence at a specific *point* in time. **Period prevalence** is the prevalence over a specified *period* of time. How do we use prevalence? As previously stated, we use it to find the magnitude or burden of a health problem in a population. We also use it to estimate the frequency of an exposure or to determine the allocation of health resources such as facilities and personnel.

$$\text{Point prevalence} = \frac{\text{Number of persons ill}}{\text{Total number in the group}} \text{ at } x \text{ point in time}$$

The **numerator** for **period prevalence** is the sum of the prevalence at the beginning of the time period in question *plus* the cases that occur during the time interval.

$$\text{Period prevalence} = \frac{\text{Number of persons ill}}{\text{Average population}} \text{ during } x \text{ time period}$$

The **denominator** for **period prevalence** is the average population over the time period in question. Sometimes we know the exact size of the population and we can use that number. But when we're considering things that are dynamic, like the exact number of patients in and out of a hospital, an average is our best method. We could calculate this average a number of different ways, but often we use the following method:

$$\frac{\text{Population at the beginning} + \text{Population at the end}}{2}$$

The period prevalence includes *everyone* (alive, dead, cured) who had the condition during the period in question.

Example: Period prevalence

Wörner et al. thought that the modern style of goalkeeping in ice hockey predisposed goalie athletes to hip and groin problems.[2]. Sweden has 128 elite ice hockey goalkeepers. Of these, 101 participated in Wörner's study designed to find out the magnitude (prevalence) of hip and groin problems among them. According to the study, 28.1 percent of goalkeepers reported a hip or groin injury in any given week, and a total of 69 percent of all goalkeepers reported a hip or groin injury at any point in the season.[3] This shows a fairly large burden of injury on goalkeepers and that we should work to reduce the number of injuries.

In this example, both the 28.1 percent of goalkeepers reporting a hip or groin injury in any given week and the 69 percent of goalkeepers reporting a hip or groin injury at any point in the season would be referred to as **period prevalence,** but the time points differ.

Example: Period prevalence and proportion

Now, let's imagine we are examining the burden of shoulder injuries in field hockey players in Metro A in 2020. On January 1, 2020, there are 1000 field hockey players, and 25 of these players come into the year with existing shoulder injuries.

Exactly 248 shoulder injuries occur to individual athletes between January 1, 2020 and December 31, 2020. On December 31, 2020, there are 1200 field hockey players in Metro A. To calculate the period prevalence, we need to add together all the shoulder injuries to create the numerator (25 + 248). We then need to create an average number of field hockey players over the year ([1000+1200]/2) as one way to account for the change over the year.

$$\text{Period prevalence} = \frac{25+248}{\left[\frac{1000+1200}{2}\right]} = \frac{273}{1100} = 0.2481$$

We could report the prevalence of shoulder injuries as 0.2481. It is an **absolute** number (a value that shows the distance from zero), so there is no context for interpreting this number. More useful to us is this number as a **relative** number (an absolute value relative to another number) such as a percentage:

$$0.2481 \times 100 = 24.81 \text{ percent}$$

Thus, 24.81 percent of field hockey players in Metro A had a shoulder injury in 2020. This number, 24.81 percent, is the **proportion** of players with a shoulder injury. Because it is a relatively large proportion, we should work with players and teams on preventing these injuries.

2.1.2 Rates

A **rate** is a **ratio** that consists of a numerator and a denominator and in which *time forms part of the denominator*. It must contain:

- Disease frequency
- Unit size of the population
- Time period during which an event occurs

When we report rates, we often use **multipliers**. You may recognize from news stories or journal articles rates being reported per 100,000 population. When we look at issues related to children or maternity, we often use 1000 as the multiplier (e.g., *per 1000 live births*). But 100,000 is the most used standard and assists us when we want to compare rates across populations.

In epidemiology we use three different forms of the rate. First is the **crude rate**. This rate is the rawest version of a rate. We have not considered any other reasons why that relationship could happen or any other related factors for the situation. It is just a simple numerator and a simple denominator.

Examples:

- Crude birth rate
- Fertility rate
- Infant mortality rate
- Fetal death rate
- Postneonatal mortality rate
- Maternal mortality rate

An example formula:

$$\text{Crude death rate} = \frac{\text{Number of deaths in a given year}}{\text{Reference population (during the midpoint of the year)}} \times 100,000$$

Example: Crude rate

In a study of student-athlete deaths in the National Collegiate Athletic Association (NCAA), Harmon et al. found that from the 2003–2004 school year though the 2012–2013 school year, there were 514 student-athlete deaths from all causes.[4] There are approximately 450,000 student-athletes in the NCAA.

$$\text{Crude death rate} = \frac{514}{450{,}000} \times 100,000 = 114.2 \text{ deaths per 100,000 NCAA student-athletes}$$

Use crude rates with caution when comparing disease frequencies between populations. Observed differences in crude rates may be the result of systematic factors (e.g., sex or age distributions) within the populations rather than true variation in rates. If this is the case, we are comparing apples to oranges. We need to make the populations as similar as possible to compare apples to apples.

If we want to compare rates across populations or even get a more accurate rate for our single population, we should do our best to use an **adjusted rate**. An adjusted rate is a measure in which statistical procedures have been applied to remove the effect of differences in composition of various populations. We can adjust using tools such as the direct method, indirect method, or regression.

The third type of rate we use is called a **specific rate**. This type of rate refers to a particular subgroup of the population defined in terms of factors such as race, age, sex, or single cause of death or illness (e.g., an age-specific death rate).

Incidence is the number of new cases of a disease that occur in a group during a certain time period. We can use incidence to help us research the etiology of disease and to provide estimates of the risk of developing disease. One way to calculate incidence is as a rate. The **incidence rate** describes the rate of development of a disease in a group over a certain time period. It has to include a numerator (number of *new* cases), denominator (population *at risk*), and time (period during which cases occur).

Example: Incidence rate

In one of our earlier examples for prevalence (see section 2.1.1), we examined shoulder injuries in field hockey players in Metro A. Remember that 248 new shoulder injuries occurred to individual athletes between January 1, 2020 and December 31, 2020. There were 1000 field hockey players in January and 25 of these players came into the year with existing shoulder injuries. If we assume that none of the players with existing injuries could be injured in January from sport, we can calculate our "at-risk" or susceptible population (1000 – 25). When calculating incidence we want to do our best to include only those who are capable of having the outcome in the denominator. If 20 of the 248 new injuries happened in January, 20 is our numerator.

$$\text{Incidence rate} = \frac{20}{1000-25} = \frac{20}{975} = 0.02051 \times 1000 = 20.51$$

We would report this as an incidence of 20.51 shoulder injuries per 1000 field hockey players in Metro A in January 2020.

2.2 Incidence Versus Prevalence

For both incidence and prevalence, we must have:

- A clear, discrete definition of the event (either the event happened or it did not)
- The time frame for the event

An event (outcome) could be the start or end of a biological process (e.g., menopause), death, remission, disease (diagnosis, start of symptoms, or relapse), or the start or end a behavior (e.g., smoking cessation).

Time, as discussed in section 1.2, can vary widely. It is query dependent and could be calendar time, age, time from study recruitment, time from an exposure (e.g., time from employment), or time from diagnosis.

Figure 2.3 displays a comparison between incidence and prevalence and examples of both. The bathtub of prevention[5] is a common graphical representation of the relationship between the two. Incidence is displayed as the water as it enters the tub. If the drain of the tub is closed, no water exits and it fills. This is similar to the relationship between incidence and prevalence. In reality, often some cases of disease do not survive or are cured; this part of the water escapes the tub. Sometimes those who are cured or are in remission have recurrences of disease and those cases are re-added to the mix. We can use them in the calculation of new cases (they are new) but also separately calculate the incidence of recurrence.

	Definition	Formula	Units	Example	Graphic representation
Incidence	All new cases in a given time (example: last year) in a population	# of new cases / # of people at risk	per unit of time	Of the 100 children at the sports camp yesterday, 20 got a sunburn. Incidence = 20/100	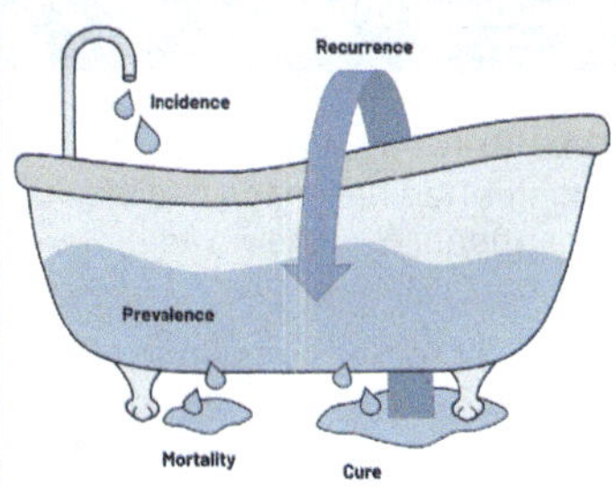
Prevalence	All cases (new + old) in a population in a given time	# of all cases / total # of people	at a point in time or during a period in time	Of the 1000 children in Town A during the summer of 2015, 50 children got a sunburn. Prevalence = 50/1000	

Figure 2.3: The bathtub of prevention.

Prevalence includes *all cases in a given time*. If you are studying a patient's survival time, mortality, or recovery time, you are interested in prevalence. Prevalence is approximately equal to the incidence of the disease times the duration (length) of the illness. What does this mean? If the duration of disease is **short** and incidence is **high**, prevalence becomes similar to incidence. Conditions that have short duration mean that cases recover rapidly or are fatal, so prevalence does not have time to build up. This is typical of certain infectious diseases such as the common cold. Conditions that have a **long** duration and a **low** incidence result in a prevalence that increases at a pace faster than incidence. This is very typical of chronic diseases. We have also come to recognize this with some infectious diseases such as HIV due to the wide availability of drug therapies and prevention strategies. If immunization programs work as intended for vaccine preventable diseases such as measles, the incidence should be low, as should prevalence. Figure 2.4 provides three scenarios in which we might calculate prevalence and what the expected outcome would be.

Possible scenarios	Corresponding outcomes for prevalence
Physical therapy shortens the time of acute hip pain for patients with bursitis.	The faster recovery time for the acute hip pain means that the prevalence of people with hip pain goes **down**. Duration of acute hip pain is short, so the number of old cases that exist at a given point is low.
Most people with untreated Rabies lyssavirus die within 10 days of symptom onset.	The fewer people that exist with the condition, the lower the numerator, so the prevalence of disease goes **down**. Duration of the infection is short, so the number of old cases that exist at a given point is low.
People who take antiretroviral drugs for HIV live a longer life.	The infection responds well to the medications, meaning that if people continue to be infected with HIV the prevalence of the disease goes **up**. The duration is long, so the numerator continues to increase.

Figure 2.4: Scenarios and outcomes for prevalence.

Incidence includes *new cases only in a given time*. This, as well as prevalence, are impacted by prevention strategies and their acceptance in the population. When we see incidence and prevalence change, we need to understand why they are changing and appropriately adjust our numbers so we can best evaluate what our next steps should be (figure 2.5).

Possible scenarios	Corresponding outcomes for incidence	Corresponding outcomes for prevalence
Nearly universal acceptance of the polio vaccination has made the disease nearly disappear from the world.	Vaccination prevents new cases, so the incidence goes **down**.	The number of cases of polio continue to drop and the number of people globally with the condition is extremely low. The prevalence also goes **down**.
A risk factor for homelessness is the lack of available and affordable housing. The hospital partners with the city to make homes available to all people in need that come into the ER.	Fewer people will be unhoused, meaning that the incidence of homelessness goes **down**.	If fewer people are unhoused, over time the prevalence of being unhoused goes **down**.
We improve the accuracy of a COVID-19 rapid test that is affordable and available to the public.	Because our test is more accurate, we will pick up more cases of the disease, so the incidence goes up.	If the incidence increases, the prevalence of ever having had the condition also goes **up**.

Figure 2.5: Scenarios and outcomes for incidence and prevalence.

Figure 2.6 summarizes various common types of prevalence and incidence and how we should interpret them. As you can see, there are at least four types of incidence that we can calculate. The difference is in how we capture the denominator and the population used. More details on when to use the different types of incidence can be found in section 2.3.

	Numerator	Denominator	Time	Interpretation
Point prevalence	All cases at that point in time (new + old)	The whole population	A single point in time (e.g., June 3, 2012 or the year 2012)	Probability (chance) of having disease at a given point in time
Period prevalence	All cases during that period (new + old)	The whole population	A particular follow-up period (e.g., after vaccine administration started)	Probability (chance) of having disease during a given period in time
Incidence rate (when you are studying a dynamic* geographic area)	New cases	People who are at risk (i.e., those susceptible to the condition) in the area or the average population of the entire geographic area	A single point or period of time	How fast disease spreads in a specific study population at a specific point in time
Incidence rate (when you are studying a dynamic* cohort of patients)	New cases	People who are at risk (i.e., those susceptible to the condition and are still in the cohort [have not dropped out])	A single point or period of time	How fast disease spreads in a specific study population at a specific point in time
Cumulative incidence (when you are studying a fixed** cohort of patients and have complete records for them all)	New cases	The initial study population	The study period	Probability (chance) of developing disease during a designated study period
Cumulative incidence (when you are studying a fixed** cohort of patients and do not have complete records for them all)	New cases	Changes depending on the time period; use of the Kaplan-Meier or Classic Life Table approach required	Points during a specific study period	Probability (chance) of developing disease at a specific point in time

*"The term "dynamic" here means that the population is steadily changing. People can continue to come in and out of the population being studied.

**The term "fixed" here means that the population is set and specific for this study. People can only leave.

Figure 2.6: Prevalence and incidence summary table.

2.3 More Details on Calculating Incidence

There are two general types of incidence: cumulative incidence and the incidence rate. The difference is how the denominator is calculated.

2.3.1 Cumulative Incidence

If we have a constrained population (we know everyone involved and we have been tracking them; e.g., a clinical trial or prospective cohort study [covered in chapter 3]), we usually calculate **cumulative incidence** because we can focus on **person-time at risk**. Cumulative incidence is a **proportion** and can only range from 0 to 1. It is an extremely precise version of incidence and requires that we have a well-defined and **closed** population (i.e., a **fixed** population).

If we have completed follow-up (meaning we have details on every subject):

$$\text{Cumulative incidence} \;=\; \frac{\text{Number of cases during follow-up}}{\text{Size of initial population}}$$

Example: Cumulative incidence

For example, if we follow a cohort of 1000 patients after their first visit to our emergency department and see that 121 return within a week for the same issue:

$$\text{Cumulative incidence} \;=\; \frac{121}{1000} = 0.121$$

The cumulative incidence of our cohort returning to the emergency department for the same issue within a week after their first visit is 0.121 or 12.1 percent.

However, the number of times you will have complete follow-up information is rare. Study subjects are often **censored**, meaning they did not complete follow-up (e.g., disappeared, moved out of the study area, left because of other health problems, died, or were recruited late in the study), meaning you will need to use either the **Kaplan-Meier method** or the **classic life table** method to calculate cumulative incidence. Cumulative incidence is also known as the **hazard** of having an outcome. It is the complement of **cumulative survival**. If we can calculate the chance of having the event, we can also calculate the chance of surviving without it. This is one place where the Kaplan-Meier method (**K-M**) and the classic life table (**CLT**) shine. They allow us to have different follow-up time for study participants, including those who started later and those who are censored.

2.3.1.1 Classic Life Table

Example: Classic life table

For example, we follow 10 postoperative orthopedic patients for one year. We are interested in finding out how long it took before the patients were cleared from rehabilitation to resume normal activities. We found that five patients completed rehabilitation before the year was over, four were censored, and one was still in rehabilitation at the end of the year.

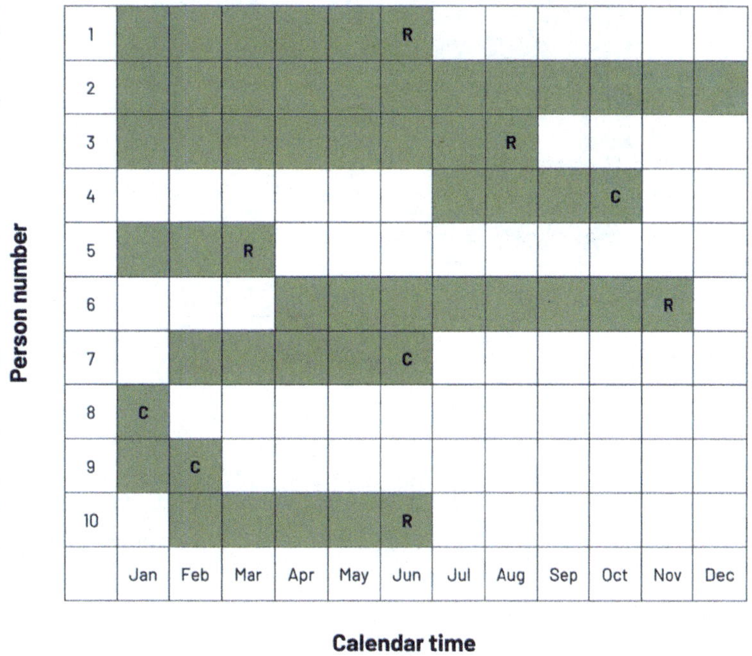

Figure 2.7: Classic life table (calendar time).

In figure 2.7, we can see a row for each of our 10 patients across the 12-month study period. We can see that some patients were enrolled in January, while others were enrolled later. Boxes that are shaded are the months the subject was in rehabilitation. The letter R denotes that the patient was released to normal activity. The letter C denotes that the patient was censored. In this example, we would calculate cumulative incidence for the patients that were released (the outcome of interest) and the cumulative survival (chance of remaining in the study without the outcome) for patients that were not released. Five patients were released and five patients were not released, so the cumulative survival is:

$$\text{Cumulative survival } = \frac{5}{10} = 0.50 \text{ or } 50 \text{ percent}$$

If we change the time scale to be months contributed to the study, we get figure 2.8.

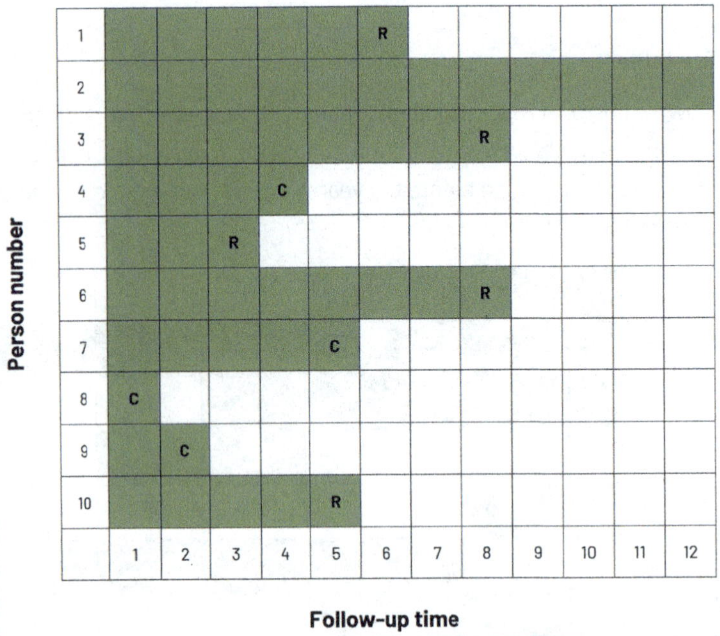

Figure 2.8: Classic life table (follow-up time).

Note that the x-axis has changed from calendar time to follow-up time. Cumulative incidence can now be calculated for each individual time point in the study. For example, if we wanted to know the incidence of being released by the end of six months (time point 6), we see that, including that time point, three patients have been released and four have been censored.

Cumulative incidence:

$$\text{Cumulative incidence}_{\text{time point t}} = \frac{\textbf{Number of individuals with the event by time point t}}{\textbf{Number at risk at baseline)}}$$

$$\text{Cumulative incidence}_{\text{time point 6}} = \frac{3}{10} = 0.30 \text{ or } 30 \text{ percent}$$

Cumulative survival:

$$\text{Cumulative survival}_{\text{time point t}} = \frac{\textbf{Number of individuals still in the study beyond time point t}}{\textbf{Number at risk at baseline)}}$$

$$\text{Cumulative survival}_{\text{time point 6}} = \frac{3}{10} = 0.30 \text{ or } 30 \text{ percent}$$

There is a problem: we lost all of the data for the people that censored at or before time point 6! Our rules tell us that we must always take into account those that have censored. If we use the CLT approach, we choose to assume that everyone that censors during the time period contributes one-half the risk in the denominator. This method assumes that censoring happens uniformly throughout the period under study.

In action, this looks like:

$$\text{Cumulative incidence}_{\text{time point t}} = \frac{\text{number of individuals with the event by time point } t}{\text{number at risk at baseline } - \frac{1}{2}\text{ (number censored)}}$$

$$\text{Cumulative incidence}_{\text{time point 6}} = \frac{3}{10-\frac{1}{2}(4)} = \frac{3}{10-2} = \frac{3}{8} = 0.375 \text{ or } 37.5 \text{ percent}$$

By the end of time point 6, 37.5 percent of patients had been released from rehabilitation to normal activity.

$$\text{Cumulative survival}_{\text{time point t}} = 1\text{-cumulative incidence}_{\text{time point t}}$$

$$\text{Cumulative survival}_{\text{time point 6}} = 1\text{-}0.375 = 0.625 \text{ or } 62.5 \text{ percent}$$

Patients remaining in the study at the end of time point 6 had a 62.5 percent chance to remain in rehabilitation past this time point.

As we can see from these results and figures 2.7 and 2.8, the probability that a patient stays in rehabilitation changes over the study. Because the chance of finishing rehabilitation or staying in rehabilitation changes over the study period (e.g., because of weather changes, changes in rehabilitation site, or changes in other medical conditions), we may need to examine this problem over multiple intervals of time. With an infectious disease such as the flu or a cold, we expect to need to calculate the cumulative incidence based on seasons of the year.

2.3.1.2 Kaplan-Meier Method

The primary difference between the classic life table and K-M methods is that in the latter we calculate the incidence and survival every time there is an event (outcome). This allows us to give all participants full credit for their time in the study.

Looking at figure 2.8, we see that patients were released from rehabilitation in month 3, month 5, month 6, and month 7. We will use this information to calculate the conditional probability of the event/survival during the study observation period. In figure 2.9, we have six columns: the time points when events happen (A); the number of patients under observation in the study at that time point (B); the number of patients with an event at that time point (C); the probability of the event occurring (conditional on it being at that time point) (D); the probability of surviving (conditional on it being at that time point) (E); and the cumulative probability of surviving to that time point (F). Note that participants are included in the denominator until after the time point when the event occurred. As an example, at time point 3, patient 5 is included in the numerator and in the denominator because that person was in the study until that point; at time point 4, the patient is no longer included in the denominator.

A	B	C	D = C/B	E = 1 - D	F
Time point	Number at risk	Number of events	Conditional probability of the event	Conditional probability of survival	Cumulative probability of survival
0	10	0	0/10 = 0.000	1 - 0.000 = 1.000	1
3	8	1	1/8 = 0.125	1 - 0.125 = 0.875	1.000 x 0.875 = 0.875
5	6	1	1/6 = 0.167	1 - 0.167 = 0.833	0.875 x 0.833 = 0.729
6	4	1	1/4 = 0.250	1 - 0.250 = 0.750	0.729 x 0.750 = 0.547
7	3	2	2/3 = 0.670	1 - .670 = 0.330	0.547 x 0.330 = 0.181

Figure 2.9: Kaplan-Meier table.

The K-M Curve (figure 2.10) is used often in clinical studies to show the cumulative survival or the cumulative incidence in graphic form. Known for its "stair step," the graph shows how the probability (y-axis) changes as time passes (x-axis). As we know from our previous figure/table as the study starts, the probability of being in rehabilitation is 100 percent. Every time a patient completes rehabilitation, the probability of being in rehabilitation ("step down" in red [top left to bottom right]) and the probability of finishing rehabilitation ("step up" in blue [bottom left to top right]) change. These two probabilities mirror each other, so display the graph that best depicts what you are trying to convey.

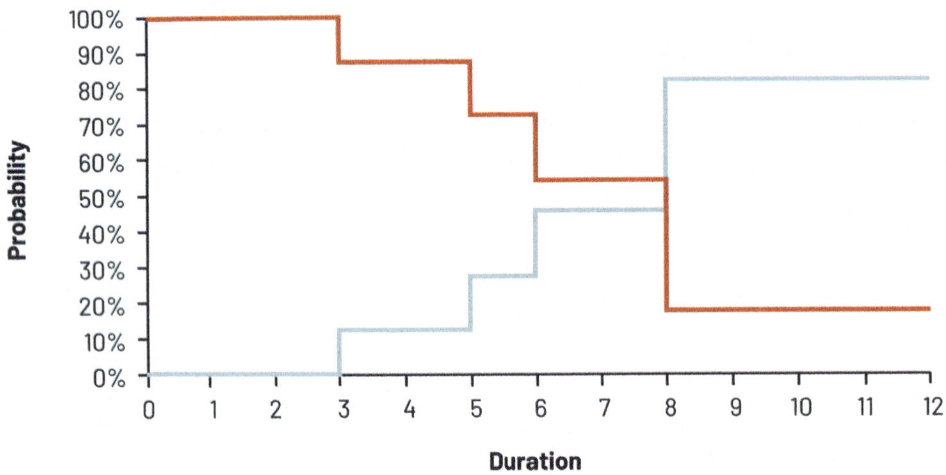

Figure 2.10: Kaplan-Meier curve.

When using this method, it is important to recognize that if your study period is long, you do not see what are called **secular trends**, meaning changes in risk over time of your study that could be attributed to something else. You also need to make sure that censoring is independent of survival (i.e., those who censor have the same prognosis as those who remain in the study). If those who censor are for some reason different from those who remain (e.g., older or sicker), the results of your study will be biased. If censored observations have a worse prognosis than those in the study, the observed survival will be greater than the real answer. If censored observations have a better prognosis than those in the study, the observed survival will be lower than the real answer. See chapter 5 for more on bias.

2.3.2 Incidence Rate

In our previous examples discussing cumulative incidence, our population was **fixed**. More often, however, we have an **open** or **dynamic** population, such as the patients in a hospital, the population of a state, or the population of students at a university. Dynamic means that people can come in and out of the population (e.g., births, deaths, migration). In this case we typically use **incidence rate** (also known as **incidence density**). The incidence rate is a ratio, but it is not a proportion. The value can be from zero to infinity.

If you have a better-defined population, like a cohort of patients from a hospital where all have a specific diagnosis coming through the emergency department and each one of them participates a different amount of time, calculating incidence using **person-time** as the denominator is the best option. If you are looking at geographical-type areas, use the **average population** as the denominator. In this instance, the formula is:

$$\text{Average population} = \frac{\text{population at the beginning of the period} + \text{population at the end of the period}}{2}$$

The average population can be calculated one of two ways.

- Method 1

  $$\text{Average population} = \frac{\text{population at the beginning of the period} + \text{population at the end of the period}}{2}$$

  Using our previous example (figure 2.9), we started with 10 people in rehabilitation and finished with 1 in rehabilitation.

  Average population = (10+1) / 2 = 11 / 2 = 5.5

  In a different example, if our town had a ski resort and the population changed several times over the year to include seasonal workers or seasonal residents, we might have more population numbers to consider. If the population during ski season was 10,000, immediately after the season was 6,000, and during the summer was 8,000, we would calculate the denominator as follows:

  Average population = (10,000 + 6,000 + 8,000) / 3 = 24,000 / 3 = 8,000

- Method 2

  Average population = population at the beginning of the period - $\frac{1}{2}$ events- $\frac{1}{2}$ censored

  Using our original example (figure 2.9), we started with 10 people in rehabilitation, 5 people had the event of interest (getting out of rehabilitation), and 4 people censored.

  Average population = $10 - \frac{1}{2}(5) - \frac{1}{2}(4) = 10 - 2.5 - 2 = 10 - 4.5 = 5.5$

  In our ski example, if 1,500 people were injured and 2,200 censored, we would calculate the denominator as follows:

  Average population = $10{,}000 - \frac{1}{2}(1{,}500) - \frac{1}{2}(2{,}200) = 10{,}000 - 750 - 1{,}100 = 10{,}000 - 1{,}850 = 8{,}150$

2.3.2.1 Person Time

Using person-time, or incidence based on how much time was contributed by participants, requires precise data from a very defined population. The denominator is calculated as how much time each person contributed to the study. For example, if we studied 5 people for 5 years, the 5 people would have contributed a total of 25 person-years to our study. If we studied 25 people for 1 year, the 25 people would have contributed a total of 25 person-years to our study. We then take this information to calculate our incidence rate (density):

$$\text{Incidence rate} = \frac{\text{number of events}}{\text{time at risk (pooled)}} \times \text{ multiplier}$$

We use person-time when we cannot determine the incidence of the event for individuals like we would with cumulative incidence but need a similar answer. We use the time unit (e.g., years, months, days) that is most relevant to the situation. For the time at risk, we assume the participant with the event provided half of the relevant time period before their outcome (e.g., if the time period is one year, the participant is assumed to have had the event at six months).

If we look at figure 2.11, we see a graphical representation of a study cohort over a four-month study period. At the beginning of the study, there are eight volleyball players on a team. We want to observe the incidence of shoulder injuries during the four-month period but only have team-level information. In the first month, one player gets a shoulder injury. In the second month, no player is injured. In the third month, four players get a shoulder injury. In the fourth month, no player is injured.

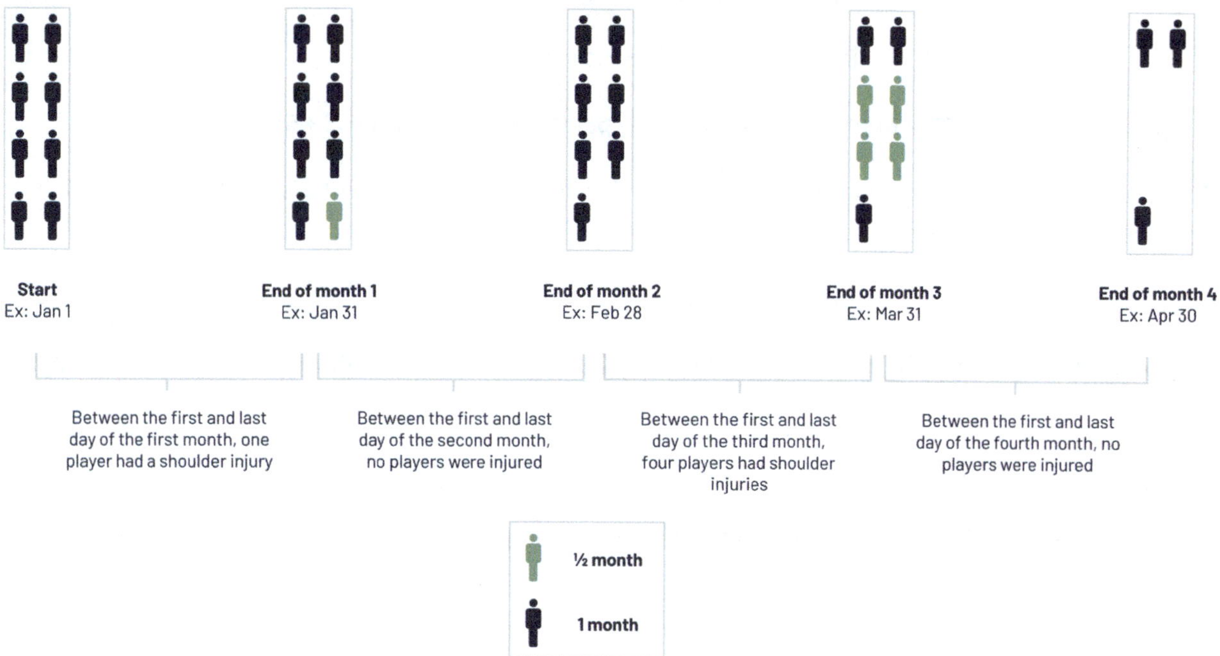

Figure 2.11: How to calculate incidence using person-time.

At the end of month 1 (*example January 1 to January 31*), the person-time contributed by the eight volleyball players is 7.5 months.

7 players uninjured → person-time = 7 x 1 = 7

1 player injured → person time = 1 x 0.5 = 0.5

The total person-time after 1 month = 7+0.5 = 7.5

The amount of person time contributed in month 2 (*example February 1 to February 28*) by the seven remaining uninjured players is seven months.

7 players uninjured → person-time = 7 x 1 = 7

The total person-time to this point is 14.5 months (7.5 + 7).

The amount of person time contributed in month 3 (*example March 1 to March 31*) by the seven remaining uninjured players is five months.

3 players uninjured → person-time = 3 x 1 = 3

4 players injured → person-time = 4 x 0.5 = 2

Total person-time added in month 3 = 3+2 = 5

The total person-time to this point is 19.5 months (14.5 + 5).

The amount of person-time contributed in month 4 (*example April 1 to April 30*) by the three remaining uninjured players is three months.

3 players uninjured → person-time = 3 x 1 = 3

The total person-time at the end of the study period (*example January 1 to April 30*) is 22.5 months (19.5 + 3).

There were a total of five injuries during the study period.

Incidence of shoulder injuries = 5 / 22.5 person-months = 0.22 injuries per person-month

or 2.67 injuries per person-year *or* 0.88 injuries per season

	Total no. of game athlete-exposures	Injuries, no.	Game injury rate per 1000 athlete-exposures	95 percent confidence interval	Total no. of practice athlete-exposures	Injuries, no.	Practice injury rate per 1000 athlete-exposures	95 percent confidence interval
Division I								
Preseason	114528	803	7.01	6.53, 7.50	4903695	35710	7.28	7.21, 7.36
In season	1963708	31883	16.24	16.06, 16.41	7305903	17502	2.4	2.36, 2.43
Postseason	89610	849	9.47	8.84, 10.11	390538	622	1.59	1.47, 1.72
Total division I	2167846	33535	15.47	15.30, 15.63	12600136	53834	4.27	4.24, 4.31
Division II								
Preseason	56590	356	6.29	5.64, 6.94	2290173	14696	6.42	6.31, 6.52
In season	1017991	13855	13.61	13.38, 13.84	3138541	7013	2.23	2.18, 2.29
Postseason	45747	388	8.48	7.64, 9.33	146101	179	1.23	1.05, 1.40
Total division II	1120328	14599	13.03	12.82, 13.24	5574815	21888	3.93	3.87, 3.98
Division III								
Preseason	115725	562	4.86	4.45, 5.26	3502829	20545	5.87	5.79, 5.95
In season	1754358	22940	13.08	12.91, 13.25	5472374	12625	2.31	2.27, 2.35
Postseason	85831	680	7.92	7.33, 8.52	252727	268	1.06	0.93, 1.19
Total division III	1955914	24182	12.36	12.21, 12.52	9227930	33438	3.62	3.58, 3.66
All divisions								
Preseason	286843	1721	6	5.72, 6.28	10696697	70951	6.63	6.58, 6.68
In season	4736057	68678	14.5	14.39, 14.61	15916818	37140	2.33	2.31, 2.36
Postseason	221188	1917	8.67	8.28, 9.05	789366	1069	1.35	1.27, 1.44
Total	5244088	72316	13.79	13.69, 13.89	27402881	109160	3.98	3.96, 4.04

Wald X^2 statistics from negative binomial model: game injury rates differed among divisions (p .01) and within season (p .01). Practice injury rates differed among divisions (p .01) and within season (p .01). Postseason sample sizes are much smaller (and have a higher variability) than preseason and in season sample sizes because only a small percentage of schools participated in the postseason tournaments in any sport and not all of those were a part of the injury Surveillance System sample. Numbers do not always sum to totals because of missing division or season information. Spring football data are not included here.

Figure 2.12: Game and practice injury rates, 15 Sports, National Collegiate Athletic Association (1988–1989 through 2003–2004).

In SRI research, person-time is often referred to as an **athlete-exposure**. Figure 2.12 is an example of the use of person-time in the NCAA Injury Surveillance Study to calculate the rates of game and practice injuries from the 1988–1989 academic year through the 2003–2004 academic year.[6] Because of the number of players and the lack of the ability to count precisely how much time each individual athlete is present for a game or a practice and how much time each spends at said event actually playing instead of not being active, being present at the event and on the roster that day counts as an exposure. Athletic-training and clinician records are often used to count the number of injuries that occurred and when they occurred for the numerator. In figure 2.12, for example, we see that for Division III sports, there were 115,725 athlete-exposures and 562 injuries during games in the preseason. Using our formula for calculating person-time and 1000 as a multiplier, we find the following:

$$\text{Game injury rate} = \frac{562}{115{,}725} \times 1000 = 0.00486 \times 1000 = 4.86 \text{ game injuries per 1000 athlete-exposures in Division III sports}$$

2.4 Dynamics of Disease

2.4.1 Demographic Transition

The **demographic transition** refers to the change in population makeup due to births, deaths, and migration. Populations move from high births and high death rates from a time before the Industrial Revolution to low birth rates and low death rates due to factors such as improved economic conditions, sanitation, and better health care. This change occurs as a population (e.g., a country) moves from being agrarian to postindustrial. The demographic transition is important in clinical medicine because as we become more dependent on industry and richer as a population, our birth rate decreases, people live longer so the death rate decreases, and the population as a whole starts to decrease in size. Figure 2.13 displays the transition using population pyramids.[7]

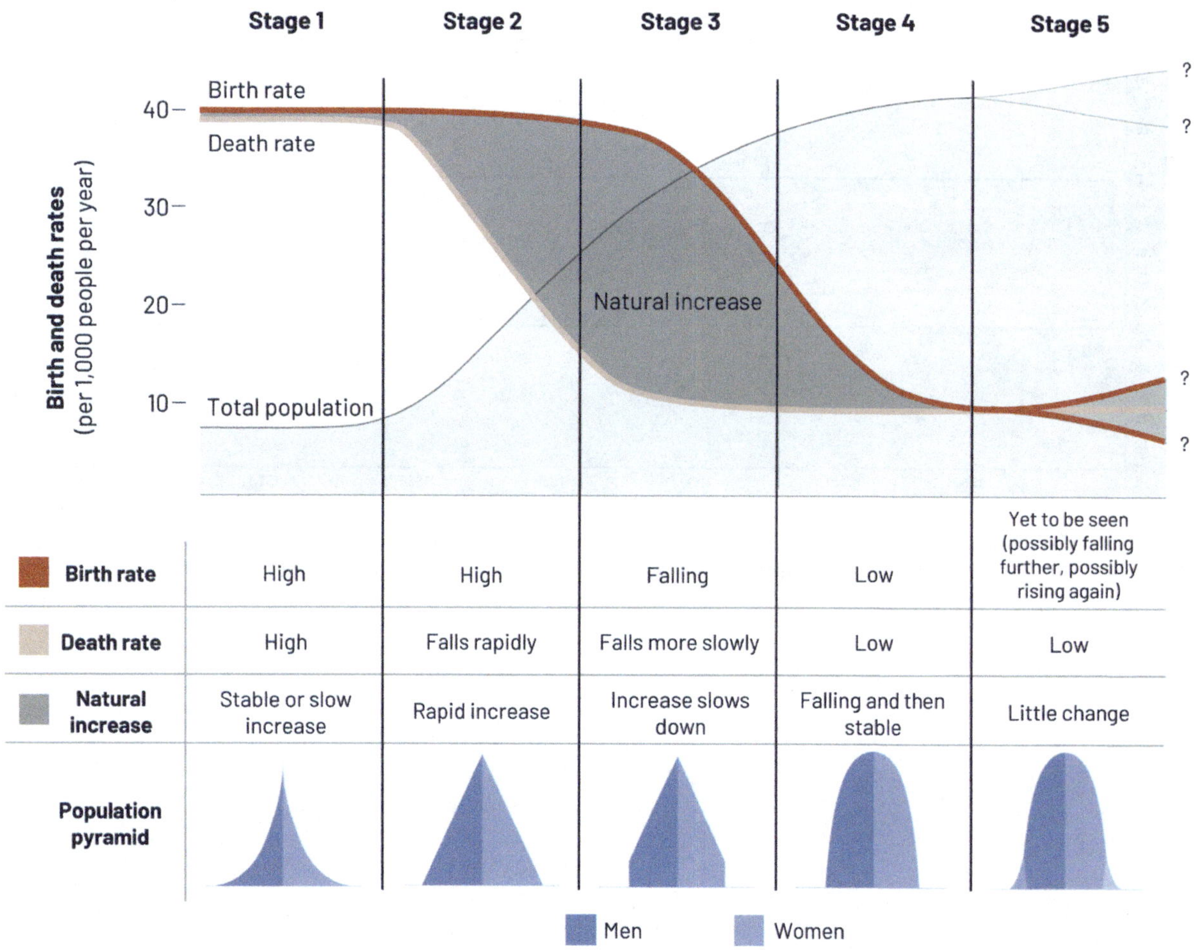

Figure 2.13: The five stages of the demographic transition. (The demographic transition is a model that describes why rapid population growth is a temporary phenomenon.)

Figure 2.14 shows how this transition has occurred in five countries. As we can see, from 1820 where the x axis starts through 2010 where it ends, the population size has increased for all countries, but each has a slightly different pattern of how births and deaths occurred. However, in all cases, the births and deaths eventually fell, and yet the overall population size remained high because people lived longer.

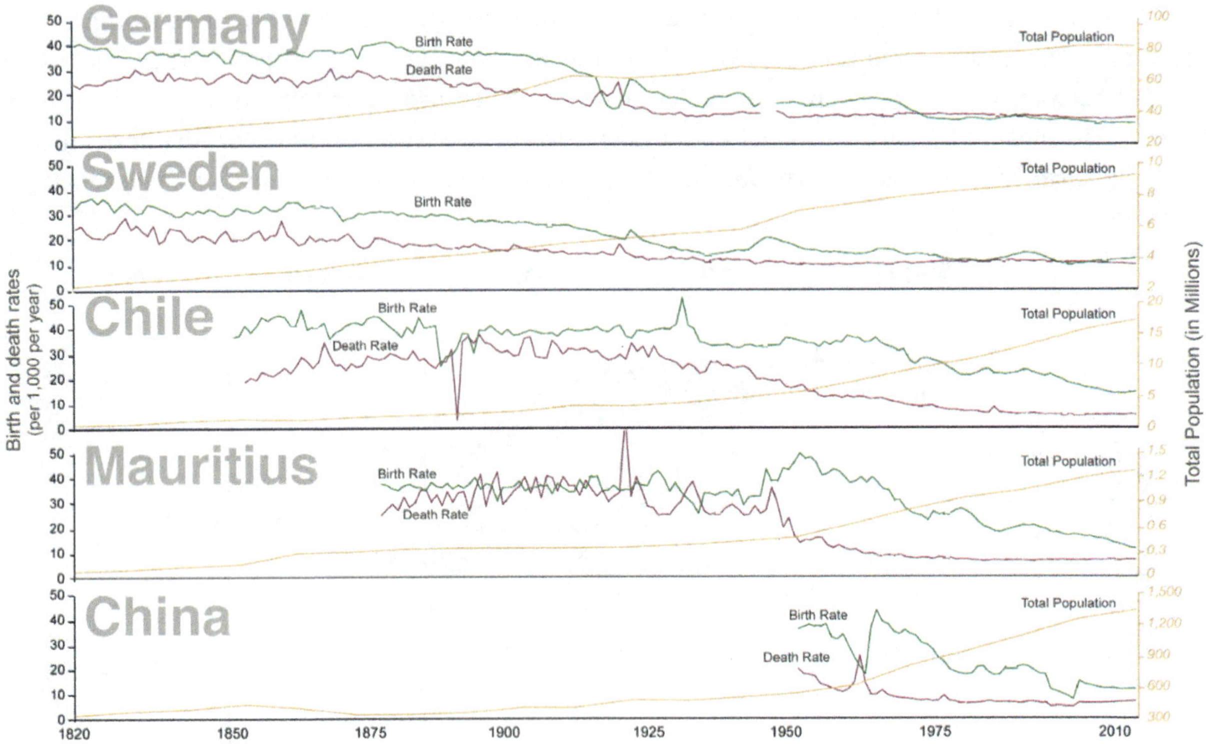

Figure 2.14: The demographic transition in five countries. (The demographic transition refers to the transition from high birth and death rates to low birth and death rates. It is shown here for five countries that achieved the transition one after the other.)

Despite overall population growth, the demographic transition also means that populations will stop growing and eventually start falling. This can be seen in figure 2.15. There are lines for the least developed countries, less developed regions, and more developed regions. We can see that from 1950 to the present day, the population growth rate for all three countries has dropped and then slightly leveled out. It is predicted that the rates will continue to drop through the end of the century.

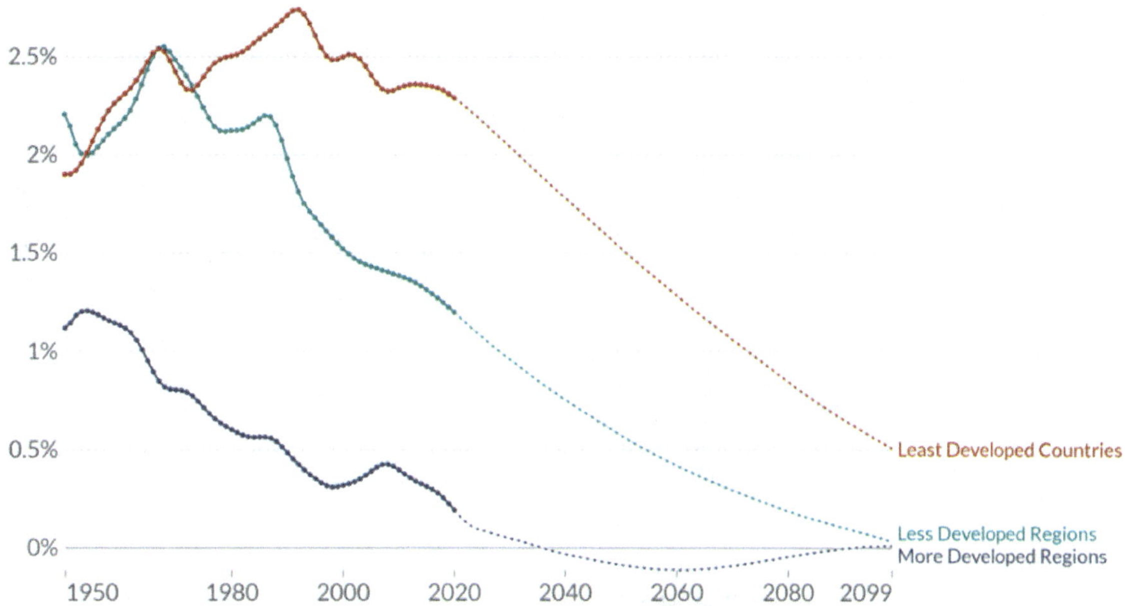

Figure 2.15: Population growth rate by level of development. Historic population growth rates by the level of development of the region, with projections to 2099 using the UN medium scenario.

2.4.2 Epidemiologic Transition

The **epidemiologic transition** is an extension of the demographic transition and refers to how as countries transition from being more agrarian to more industrial, the causes of their deaths tend to change as well. In more agricultural societies and when populations have high rates of births and deaths, the causes of death tend to be infectious diseases and complications from reproduction. As populations become more industrial and even postindustrial, the advent of better sanitation, health care, transportation, and so on allows for improvements in care to reduce the burden of infectious diseases and reproductive outcomes. As people live longer, they become more susceptible to noncommunicable diseases and injury such as heart disease and falls. The originator of the epidemiologic transition theory,[8] Dr. Abdel Omran, has published in length about this idea (see figures 2.16 and 2.17).

In figure 2.16, we can see all of the dynamics that feed into the epidemiologic transition and how it is built on top of the demographic transition.

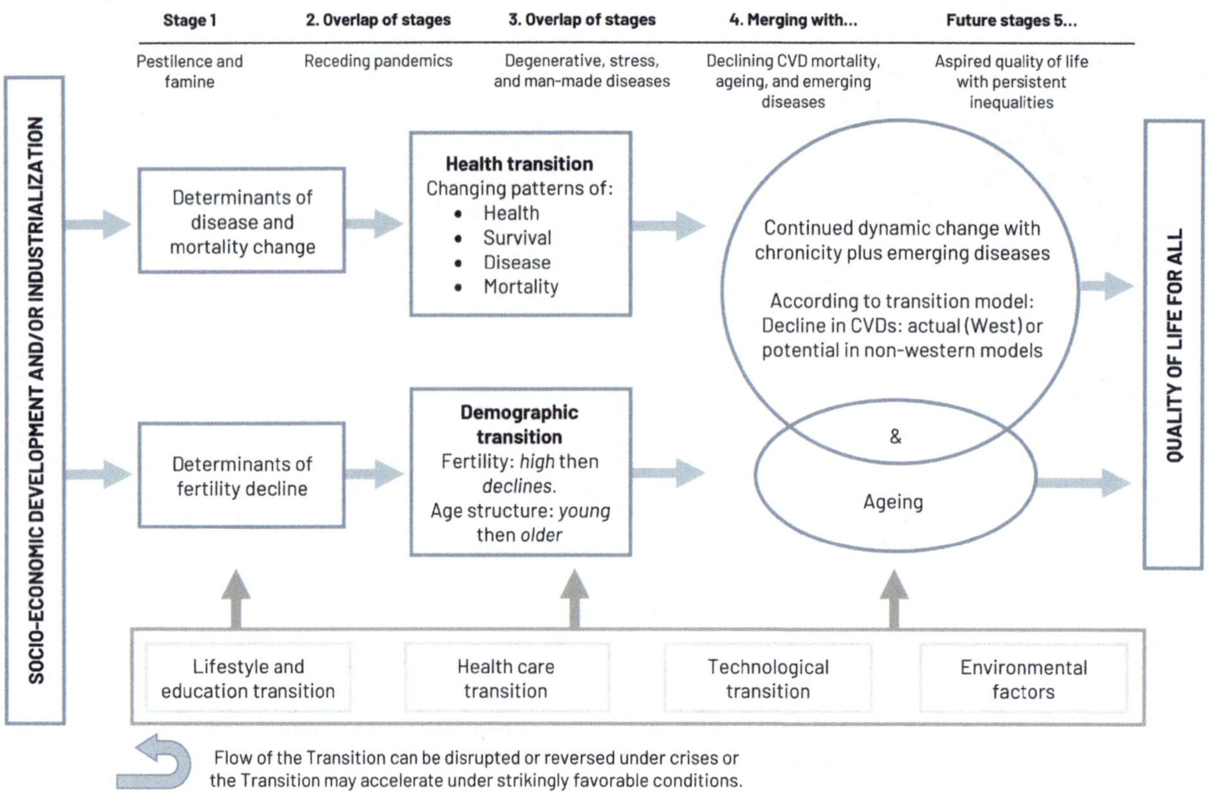

Figure 2.16: The epidemiologic transition dynamics.

In figure 2.17, we can see the movement of the preventable disease burden over time and how this impacts what we see in the clinical space.

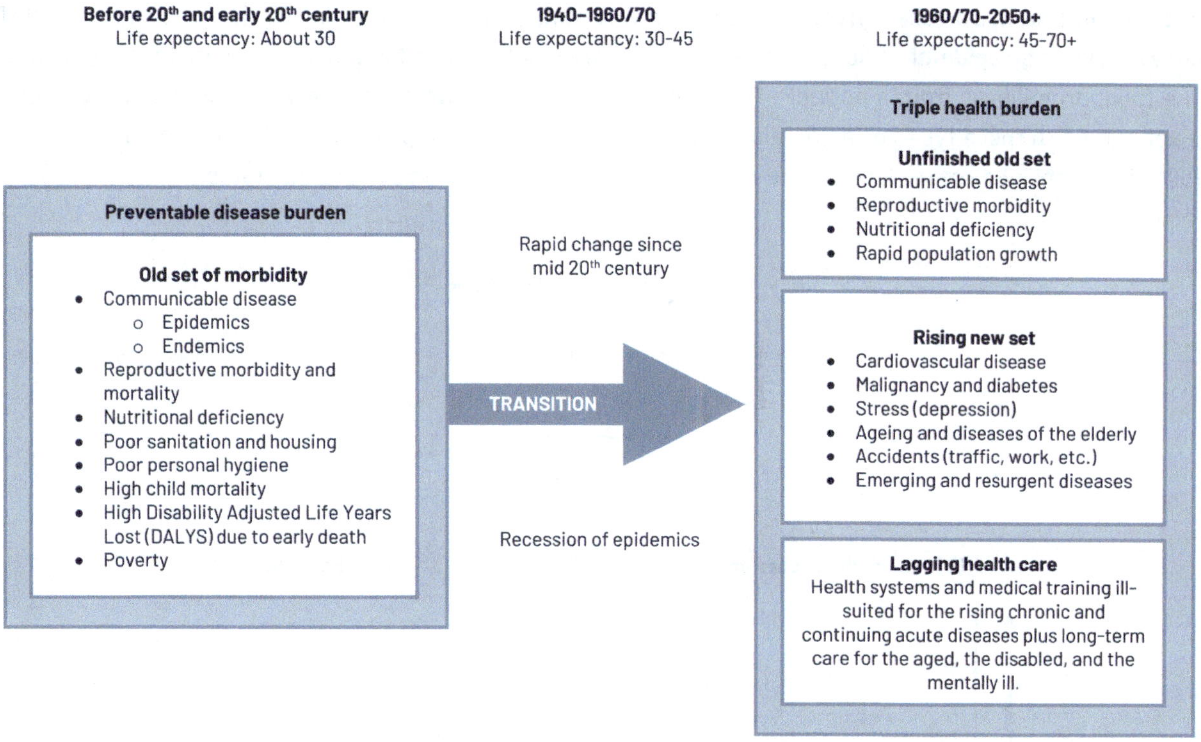

Figure 2.17: Transition stages in the developing countries.

2.4.3 Epidemic Curve

One mechanism used to examine disease in populations, particularly infectious diseases, is the **epidemic curve** (epi curve). An epi curve is a visual display of the onset of illness among cases associated with an outbreak.

You can learn a lot about an outbreak from an epi curve,[9] such as:

- The outbreak's time trend; that is, the distribution of cases over time
- Outliers; that is, cases that stand apart from the overall pattern
- General sense of the outbreak's magnitude
- Inferences about the outbreak's pattern of spread
- The most likely time period of exposure

In an epi curve, the x-axis represents the time frame of interest. Depending on the condition, this time frame might need to be minutes, hours, days, weeks, months, or even years. The y-axis is the incidence of cases of disease. This scale depends on how many cases exist. In figure 2.18, example B shows what we might see if we plot a disease that occurs sporadically, like Creutzfeldt-Jakob Disease. Example C shows what we might see with an **endemic** disease. In the United States, an example of an endemic disease is influenza. Example D shows us what an **epidemic** disease that is spread from a single source looks like if we were to plot the cases like foodborne illness from a potluck. This is different from **epidemic** disease with a **propagating** source (Example E). In these types of epidemics, the initial wave of disease propagates (i.e., is the source of) the following cases of disease. An example would be a measles outbreak in the United States.

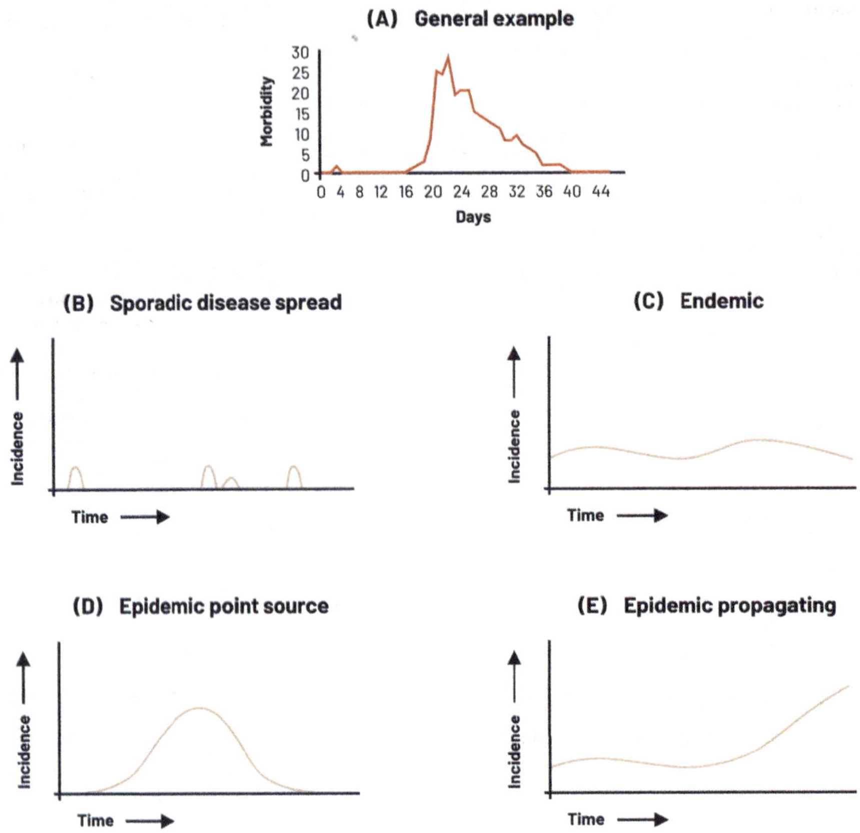

Figure 2.18: Examples of epidemic curves.

Figure Descriptions

Figure 2.2: Triangle representing ratios with consideration of population size and strength of evidence. Size of population affected is larger as triangle widens at bottom. Strength of evidence is weaker as triangle widens at bottom. From top to bottom. 1:1 (mortality=2645), 25:1 (hospitalizations=67301), 363:1 (emergency room visits=959278), 73:1 (treatment by non-ED physicians=192200), 295:1 (functional impairment=1310500), 729:1 (number of injuries causing functional impairment*=1928000), 3646:1 (total population 12 and older=9642760). Return to figure 2.2.

Figure 2.7: Boxed table with calendar time on x-axis and person number on y-axis. Each row is shaded and labeled with respect to when the person was enrolled, censored, or released from (completed) rehabilitation. Across twelve months, shading of each person's participation is staggered based on different enrollment and release times. Return to figure 2.7.

Figure 2.8: Boxed table with follow up time on x-axis and person number on y-axis. Each row is shaded and labeled with respect to when the person was censored or released from (completed) rehabilitation. Exact enrollment time in this table is negligible. Follow-up time simply tracks the total length (in months) of participation in rehabilitation. Return to figure 2.8.

Figure 2.10: Graph with duration (0-12) on the x-axis and probability on the y-axis. A red line shows originates at 100% at duration 0 and decreases over duration, ending at the bottom right. A blue line starts at 0% at duration 0 and increases over duration, ending at the top right. The lines intersect at duration 8. Return to figure 2.10.

Figure 2.11: At start (Ex: Jan 1), 8 people in figure are all shaded black. Between the first and last day of the first month, one player had a shoulder injury. At end of month 1 (Ex: Jan 31), 1 of these people is shaded green, indicating a new case. Between the first and last day of the second month, no players were injured. At end of month 2 (Ex: Feb 28), 7 people are shaded black. Between the first and last day of the third month, four players had shoulder injuries. At end of month 3 (Ex: Mar 31), 3 people are shaded black and 4 people are shaded green. Between the first and last day of the fourth month, no players were injured. At end of month 4 (Ex: Apr 30), the 3 remaining people are shaded black, and are uninjured (no new cases). Return to figure 2.11.

Figure 2.13: Stages 1 through 5, from left to right, depicting birth and death rates for each stage. In Stage 1, birth and death rates are high and equivalent. In Stage 2, birth rates are higher than death rates, which are rapidly decreasing. In Stage 3, birth rates are rapidly falling and death rates are more steadily declining. In Stage 4, birth rates are falling but death rates have stabilized. In Stage 5, there is little change. Across Stages 1-4, the total population increases, until Stage 5, in which total population may rise or fall. Natural increase is shaded gray and depicts the gap between birth and death rates. Below demographic transition model, five population pyramids with men on the left half and women on the right half, depicting the spread of the population across sexes in each stage. Stage 1-3 population pyramids are triangular, and round out at Stage 4 and 5. Return to figure 2.13.

Figure 2.14: Graph with years from 1820 to 2010 on x-axis, birth and death rates (per 1,000 per year) on left y-axis, and total population (in millions) on right y-axis. From top to bottom, countries included are Germany, Sweden, Chile, Mauritius, and China. For each country, total population is represented by a yellow line, birth rate by a green line, and death rate by a red line. Total population increases over time in all 5 countries, but the transitions are represented by the interaction between birth and death rates which varies from country-to-country. In Germany, Birth and death rates were above the total population from 1820 to around the 1900s, after which the death rate line falls below the total population, as does birth rates around 1912. Both the birth and death rates remain below the total population line for the remainder of the time. Return to figure 2.14.

Figure 2.15: Years on x-axis from 1950 to 2099. Growth rate expressed as percentage on y-axis from 0% to 2.5%. Least developed countries and less developed regions have a consistently higher population growth rate than more developed regions. All 3 population growth rates are predicted to decline drastically by 2099. Return to figure 2.15.

Figure 2.16: Flow chart with epidemiological stages and transitions. Stage 1 is indicated by Pestilence and famine,

2 is Overlap of stages with receding pandemics, 3 is Overlap of stages with degenerative, stress and man-made diseases, 4 is Merging with declining CVD mortality, ageing, and emerging diseases, and 5 is Future stages with aspired quality of life with persistent inequalities. On the left, the flow chart begins with socio-economic development and/or industrialization followed by two key epidemiological transition models. On the top, Health transition is preceded by determinants of disease and morality changes, which is part of the lifestyle and education transition. Health transition is defined as changing patterns of health, survival, disease, and mortality. Then, as part of technological transitions and environmental factors, Health transition moves towards continued dynamic change with chronicity plus emerging diseases, and decline in CVDs in West (actual) or non-western models (potentially). On the bottom, Demographic transition is preceded by determinants of fertility decline, which is part of the lifestyle and education transition. Demographic transition is characterized by high fertility followed by decline, as well as changes in age structure from young to old. In technological transition and influence from environmental factors, this shifts towards ageing. Both Health transition and Demographic transitions affect the quality of life for all, the final arrow in the flow chart. Flow of the Transition can be disrupted or reversed under crises or the Transition may accelerate under strikingly favorable conditions. Return to figure 2.16.

Figure 2.17: Timeline with three time periods. First period: Before 20th and early 20th century when life expectancy was about 30. A time of preventable disease burden. Old set of morbidity: communicable disease (epidemics and endemics), reproductive morbidity and mortality, nutritional deficiency, poor sanitation and housing, poor personal hygiene, high child mortality, high Disability Adjusted Life Years Lost (DALYS) due to early death, and poverty. Second time period: 1940-1960/70 when life expectancy was 30-45. A transitional period with rapid change since the mid 20th century and a recession of epidemics. Third time period: 1960/70-2050+ when life expectancy is 45-70+. A time of triple health burden. 1: Unfinished old set (communicable disease, reproductive morbidity, nutritional deficiency, rapid population growth). 2: Rising new set (cardiovascular disease, malignancy and diabetes, stress/depression, ageing and diseases of the elderly, accidents from traffic, work, etc., emerging and resurgent diseases). 3: Lagging health care (health systems and medical training ill-suited for the rising chronic and continuing acute diseases plus long-term care for the ages, the disabled, and the mentally ill). Return to figure 2.17.

Figure 2.18: 5 graphs with time on the x-axis and incidence on the y-axis. A: general example with days on x-axis and morbidity on y-axis (incidence is low until mid-way, incidence spikes very high and then slowly over time decreases). B: sporadic disease spread (four random incidences over time, all with a low incidence value). C: endemic (over time incidence rises and falls slightly but is never at zero and is never very high). D: epidemic point source (standard bell curve; incidence rises in the middle and tapers off left and right). E: epidemic propagating (over time incidence rises and falls slightly and then at a certain time continues to rise and never fall). Return to figure 2.18.

Figure References

Figure 2.2: Deaths to injury severity ratio example. Kindred Grey. 2022. Adapted under fair use from Sahai VS, Ward MS, Zmijowskyj T, Rowe BH. Quantifying the iceberg effect for injury: Using comprehensive community health data [published correction appears in Can J Public Health. 2006 Jan-Feb;97(1):34]. Can J Public Health. 2005;96(5):328-332. DOI:10.1007/BF03404025

Figure 2.3: The bathtub of prevention. Graphic by Kindred Grey. 2022. CC BY 4.0. Table data adapted under fair use from USMLE First Aid, Step 1.

Figure 2.6: Prevalence and incidence summary table. Adapted under fair use from table 2 of An Introduction to Veterinary Epidemiology by Mark Stevenson (2008).

Figure 2.7: Classic life table (calendar time). Kindred Grey. 2022. CC BY 4.0.

Figure 2.8: Classic life table (follow-up time). Kindred Grey. 2022. CC BY 4.0.

Figure 2.10: Kaplan-Meier curve. Kindred Grey. 2022. CC BY 4.0.

Figure 2.11: How to calculate incidence using person-time. Kindred Grey. 2022. CC BY 4.0.

Figure 2.12: Game and practice injury rates, 15 sports, National Collegiate Athletic Association (1988-1989 through 2003-2004). Data from Hootman JM, Dick R, Agel J. Epidemiology of collegiate injuries for 15 sports: Summary and recommendations for injury prevention initiatives. J Athl Train. 2007;42(2):311-319.

Figure 2.13: The five stages of the demographic transition. Kindred Grey. 2022. CC BY-SA 4.0. Adapted from Roser M. Demographic-TransitionOWID, from WikimediaCommons (CC BY-SA 4.0).

Figure 2.14: The demographic transition in five countries. Roser M. CC BY 4.0. From OurWorldinData.

Figure 2.15: Population growth rate by level of development. Roser M, Ritchie H, Ortiz-Ospina E, Rodés-Guirao L. World Population Growth. 2013. CC BY 4.0. Published online at OurWorldInData.org.

Figure 2.16: The epidemiologic transition dynamics. Kindred Grey. 2022. CC BY-NC-SA 3.0 IGO. Adapted from Omran AR. The epidemiologic transition theory revisited thirty years later. World Health Stat Q. 1998;53 (2, 3, 4), 99-119. World Health Organization. (CC BY-NC-SA 3.0 IGO)

Figure 2.17: Transition stages in the developing countries. Kindred Grey. 2022. CC BY-NC-SA 3.0 IGO. Adapted from Omran AR. The epidemiologic transition theory revisited thirty years later. World Health Stat Q. 1998;53 (2, 3, 4), 99 -119. World Health Organization. (CC BY-NC-SA 3.0 IGO)

Figure 2.18: Examples of epidemic curves. Kindred Grey. 2022. CC BY 4.0.

Notes

1. Sorenson SB. Gender disparities in injury mortality: Consistent, persistent, and larger than you'd think. *Am J Public Health*. 2011;101(Suppl 1):S353-358.
2. Wörner T, Clarsen B, Thorborg K, Eek F. Elite ice hockey goalkeepers have a high prevalence of hip and groin problems associated with decreased sporting function: A single-season prospective cohort study. Orthop J Sports Med. 2019;7(12) https://doi.org/10.1177/2325967119892586
3. Wörner T, Clarsen B, Thorborg K, Eek F. Elite ice hockey goalkeepers have a high prevalence of hip and groin problems associated with decreased sporting function: A single-season prospective cohort study. Orthop J Sports Med. 2019;7(12) https://doi.org/10.1177/2325967119892586
4. Harmon KG, Asif IM, Maleszewski JJ, et al. Incidence, cause, and comparative frequency of sudden cardiac death in National Collegiate Athletic Association athletes: A decade in review. *Circulation*. 2015;132(1):10-19.
5. Bhopal RS. *Concepts of Epidemiology: Integrating the Ideas, Theories, Principles, and Methods of Epidemiology*. 2nd ed. Oxford University Press; 2008. https://doi.org/10.1093/acprof:oso/9780199543144.001.0001
6. Hootman JM, Dick R, Agel J. Epidemiology of collegiate injuries for 15 sports: Summary and recommendations for injury prevention initiatives. *J Athl Train*. 2007;42(2):311-319.
7. Roser M, Ritchie H, Ortiz-Ospina E. World population growth. https://ourworldindata.org/population-growth. Published 2013. Accessed 2022.
8. Omran AR. The epidemiologic transition: A theory of the epidemiology of population change. Milbank Mem Fund Q. 1971;49(4):509-538.
9. Centers for Disease Control and Prevention. Quick-Learn Lesson: Create an Epi Curve. https://www.cdc.gov/training/quicklearns/createepi/index.html. Published 2021. Accessed September 12, 2023.

3. STUDY DESIGNS

3.1 Measurement Through Study

There are two primary categories of study designs (figure 3.1), and the primary difference between the two is whether or not we *control* the study factors.

In **observational** studies, we *do not* manipulate any study factors and *do not* randomize. We observe what happens in a particular group of people—for example, factory workers, children in a preschool, or patients seen in a clinic for primary care. When we say *manipulate*, we do not mean that we make things up. What we do mean is that we can set the parameters of the study (i.e., control study factors) such as who gets the exposure (e.g., a medication) or who does not (e.g., the placebo or standard of care) in order to see causal effects, if they exist between an exposure and an outcome. When we do this, it is called an **experimental** study.

In **experimental** studies, we do control factors and often use randomization to create fairly perfect conditions to see the influence of an exposure on an outcome. For example, we might enroll some cancer patients in a trial to see how a new medication works, or we might test how different the health is in communities with fluoridated water compared to those without fluoridated water. Randomization means that we use some sort of objective criteria to put study participants in whatever groups we establish for our study. For example, we may have one group that gets a sugar pill (i.e., a placebo), one group that gets the standard of care, and one group that gets the drug we are testing. In this scenario, we might assign patients to a group based on the order in which they come to the clinic. We might also choose to assign all patients a number and randomly allocate them to a group using a random number generator. No matter the assignation, we use an objective method to put patients in a study group. This helps us reduce the chance of a biased study result.

As you consider each study design, pay attention to these details:

- Number of observations made
- Directionality of exposure
- Data collection methods
- Timing of data collection
- Unit of observation
- Availability of subjects

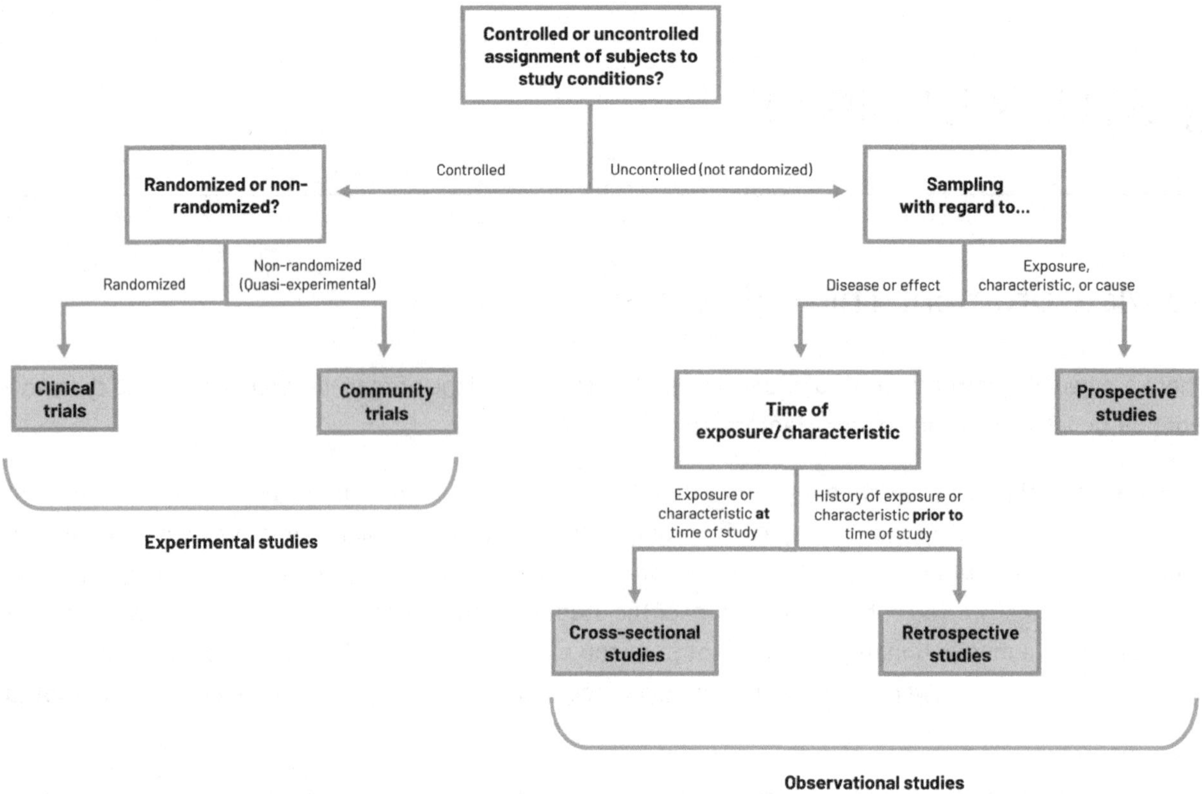

Figure 3.1: Overview of study designs.

All study designs are not created to be equal, but each has a specific purpose. Each study design helps us move closer to an understanding of causality (section 1.2). As you move from *in-vitro* studies to *meta-analyses* (figure 3.2), you can see that the evidence each study design provides becomes stronger. It does not mean the designs at the top are weaker or useless, they just provide a different type of evidence. Though there is a general consensus about how valid or strong the evidence is from any particular type of study, the evidence from each design builds on the others.

Study types	
In-vitro	Least strong information. Just as important as the study types below.*
Animal research	
Anecdotes, opinions, ideas	
Case reports, case series	
Ecologic study	
Cross-sectional	
Case control	
Cohort	
Community trials	
Randomized control trials (RCT)	
Systematic reviews	
Meta-analyses	Strongest information. Just as important as the study types above.*
*All study types are important and each level builds on the ones before it.	

Figure 3.2: How much can we rely on the answers from your study when determining the etiology (cause) of disease or conditions?

Example: Types of study designs

What happens when we approach the same topic and question with different study designs? Let's find out using osteoarthritis as an example.

- In vitro: In vitro models for the study of osteoarthritis
- Animal: Animal models of osteoarthritis: classification, update, and measurement of outcomes
- Opinion: Current opinion: where are we in our understanding and treatment of osteoarthritis?
- Case report: The effect of knee resizing illusions on pain and swelling in symptomatic knee osteoarthritis: a case report
- Cross-sectional: Is There an Association Between a History of Running and Symptomatic Knee Osteoarthritis? A Cross-Sectional Study From the Osteoarthritis Initiative
- Case control: A case-control study to investigate the relation between low and moderate levels of physical activity and osteoarthritis of the knee using data collected as part of the Allied Dunbar National Fitness Survey
- Cohort: Running does not increase symptoms or structural progression in people with knee

osteoarthritis: data from the osteoarthritis initiative

- RCT: Ultrasound-Guided Injection of Platelet-Rich Plasma and Hyaluronic Acid, Separately and in Combination, for Hip Osteoarthritis: A Randomized Controlled Study
- Systematic review: Is Participation in Certain Sports Associated With Knee Osteoarthritis? A Systematic Review
- Meta-analysis: Is Participation in Certain Sports Associated With Knee Osteoarthritis? A Systematic Review

In the real world, study designs are not always clearly distinguishable from each other. There often is overlap such as that seen in the nested case-control, cross-sectional case-control, and case-cohort study designs.

3.2 Study Designs

Beyond the measures presented in chapter 2, epidemiologic studies allow us to create and compare measures across individuals and groups. Because we are really examining the relationship between factors, exposures, and outcomes, we call the majority of these **measures of association**. Figures 3.3 and 3.4 lay out the different types of studies and some overview details about them. The rest of this chapter is dedicated to explaining and discussing **temporality**, **measures of association**, **measures of effect**, and **sampling**.

Figure 3.3 describes five types of observational study designs: case series, ecologic studies, cross-sectional studies, case-control studies, and cohort studies. From left to right, the designs are listed in order of the strength of their evidence (weakest to strongest).

Details	**Observational designs (in order of strength)**				
	Case series	**Ecologic**	**Cross-sectional**	**Case control**	**Cohort**
Also known as	Case study	Correlational study	Prevalence study	Case-referent study	Follow-up study
Descriptive or analytic?	Descriptive	Primarily descriptive	Descriptive	Analytic	Analytic
Can temporality be determined?	No	No	No	No	Yes
Unit of observation	Individual	Group	Individual	Individual	Individual
Major uses of the design/ What is the design good for?	Describe interesting cases of disease, injury, or other health issues.	Test or develop etiologic hypotheses (hypotheses about the population). Create hypotheses about causation or identify methods of prevention.	Present the burden of disease, injury, or other health issues (morbidity or mortality). Generate hypotheses. Supports planning health services.	Outbreaks, studying diseases of low prevalence, testing hypotheses.	Studying etiology, providing direct measures of risk, testing hypotheses, showing temporal relationships, looking at rare exposures.
What measures or measures of association are used with the design?	None	Correlation, chi-square	Prevalence estimates, prevalence rate ratio (AKA prevalence relative risk)	Odds ratio	Relative risk (most often), odds ratio (sometimes)
Formula	N/A	Depends on the design	$\mathrm{PRR} = \frac{\frac{A}{A+B}}{\frac{C}{C+D}}$ (Uses prevalence not incidence like the RR)	$\mathrm{OR} = \frac{AD}{BC}$ This cross-product ratio is the derivative of: $\frac{\frac{A}{A+C}/\frac{C}{A+C}}{\frac{B}{B+D}/\frac{D}{B+D}}$	$\mathrm{RR} = \frac{\frac{A}{A+B}}{\frac{C}{C+D}}$ (Direct Measurement of Risk) $\mathrm{OR} = \frac{AD}{BC}$ (Indirect Measurement of Risk) This cross-product ratio is the derivative of: $\frac{\frac{A}{A+B}/\frac{B}{A+B}}{\frac{C}{C+D}/\frac{D}{C+D}}$

Details	Observational designs (in order of strength)				
	Case series	**Ecologic**	**Cross-sectional**	**Case control**	**Cohort**
Advantages	Able to share information with others to then develop hypotheses or plan studies.	Quick and easy to conduct. Inexpensive.	Sometimes quick and relatively easy to conduct (if using secondary vs primary data). Inexpensive.	Great with rare outcomes. Cheap, efficient. Can be completed rather quickly.	Great with rare exposures. Can show temporal relationships between exposure and disease retrospectively, prospectively, or a combination of the two.
Disadvantages	Not enough details to make decisions for treatment.	Ecologic fallacy. Imprecise measurement.	Not good for rare diseases. Shouldn't be used for etiologic studies.	Not good for rare exposures. Cannot provide a direct measure of risk. Recall bias.	Can cost a lot of money and take a lot of time to complete. Difficult to execute. Selection bias. Not good for rare diseases.
Example	We had five patients with hallucinations after taking NSAID A that is not known for causing hallucinations. We will describe their clinical presentation here.	The rate of premature births decreased in West Virginia when Medicaid was expanded.	The prevalence of high adiposity increased in New Mexico during the COVID-19 pandemic amongst people 60 to 65 years of age that were retired.	People that worked in grocery stores during the first four months of the COVID-19 pandemic were more likely to be hospitalized with COVID-19 than the general population.	Soldiers that entered boot camp in 1980 and stayed in the military for 20 years had a higher risk of osteoarthritis at 60 than soldiers that entered at the same time and stayed in the military less than 7 years.

PRR: Prevalence Rate Ratio
OR: Odds Ratio
RR: Relative Risk

Figure 3.3: Epidemiological study designs.

Figure 3.4 describes two types of experimental study designs: community trials and clinical trials.

Details	Experimental designs	
	Community trial	**Clinical trial**
Also known as	Community intervention study	RCT
Descriptive or analytic?	Analytic	Analytic
Can temporality be determined?	Yes	Yes
Unit of observation	Community	Individual
Major uses of the design/ What is the design good for?	Useful for seeing how effective community-level interventions are, evaluating policies, or implementing healthier behaviors in the community.	Useful for testing efficacy of new medications, therapies, treatments, or preventative methods (such as vaccines). If a multiphase trial, the steps are: Can **I swim**? Phase 0: **Initial** efficacy work (pharmacodynamics and pharmacokinetics) Phase I: **Safety** assessment Phase II: Does it **work**? Phase III: Does it lead to any **improvement** in the condition? Phase IV: Are there any issues that require us to pull it off the **market**?
Formula	Depends on the design	Depends on the design
Advantages	Randomization of communities. Researchers can sometimes manipulate the exposure. Can establish causality.	Randomization of subjects. Can manipulate exposure. Can control everything else. Can set up as a cross-over trial (same group of participants serves as both the cases and the controls). Can establish causality.
Disadvantages	Hard to control everything such as people moving in and out of the study area. Impossible to make everyone in the area participate.	The fact everything is controlled means it is uncertain whether it will work the same way in the real world.
Example	Communities with fluoridated water have better oral health outcomes than communities without fluoridated water.	Drug B is more efficacious at reducing atrial fibrillation than standard of care during a phase III trial.

Figure 3.4: Community trials and clinical trials.

One tool that is used to calculate a number of epidemiological measures is the 2×2 table (figure 3.5). This table is repeated many times in the following text. The primary columns represent the presence (e.g., outcome +) or absence (e.g., outcome –) of the outcome or event of interest (e.g., ACL injury). The primary rows represent the presence (e.g., exposed +) or absence (e.g., exposed –) of the exposure of interest (e.g., being hit). In this example table we also show the total number of those exposed and the total number of those with the outcome. These totals are sometimes needed for different calculations.

	Outcome (+)	**Outcome (-)**	Total outcome
Exposed (+)	A	B	A + B
Exposed (-)	C	D	C + D
Total exposed	A + C	B + D	A + B + C + D

Figure 3.5: Example 2×2 table.

The letters A, B, C, and D represent the number of observations that meet different criteria.

A = The count of observations that have both the outcome and the exposure

B = The count of observations that have the exposure but not the outcome

C = The count of observations that have the outcome but not the exposure

D = The count of observations that have neither the outcome nor the exposure

Using this same logic, the sum of A and B gives us the total number of observations with the exposure and the sum of C and D gives us the total number of observations without the exposure. The sum of A and C gives us the total number of observations with the outcome and the sum of B and D gives us the total number of observations without the outcome.

3.3 Temporality

In order to establish causality, it is important to be able to establish a temporal—or time—relationship between factors. As seen in figures 3.3 and 3.4, all studies are not good at measuring temporality. All studies also are not intended to measure temporality. Studies such as cohort studies or RCTs are the most used when trying to answer questions such as "Did the chicken come first or did the egg?" [Answer to that question![1]]. Figure 3.6 displays at what point in time data collection for different studies starts, the directionality of data collection, and the minimum number of time points captured by the study. For example, in a cross-sectional study all data is captured at the same point in time (the present day) and shows what is happening right now. Cross-sectional studies can be thought of as a snapshot in time, and the time period could vary from something such as a patient's last visit to patient outcomes over the last year. Because all questions get asked at once and typically involve recalling events from the past, we cannot determine temporality. A cross-sectional study can, however, give us a great perspective about the prevalence of a particular health issue. A retrospective cohort study, on the other hand, starts in the present day but looks backwards to capture information from the past. Oftentimes, there can be confusion about the difference between a retrospective cohort study and a case-control study. Even in a retrospective cohort study, our goal is to determine if a known exposure leads to a disease, such as when we are trying to determine whether playing football leads to developing chronic traumatic encephalopathy (CTE). We have information about the population both before and after diagnosis, which allows us to observe whether the exposure led to the disease. In a case-control study, we are looking to find what exposures could have led to known disease. It is most often used when we need an answer quickly, such as in an outbreak; for example, what caused an outbreak of ringworm in wrestlers. While we start with people we know have the outcome, we have to determine what possible exposures are of interest and then narrow down which one had the higher probability of causing the outcome. We cannot definitively determine temporality. One of the main differences between a prospective cohort study and a randomized control trial is that instead of seeing the natural course of exposure (e.g., choice to smoke or not smoke), we instead randomly allocate participants into our study groups—we choose for them. This means we may give one group the standard of care for an ankle injury and give the other group a new cryotherapy plus standard of care to see the effect the cryotherapy has on the outcome of the injury.

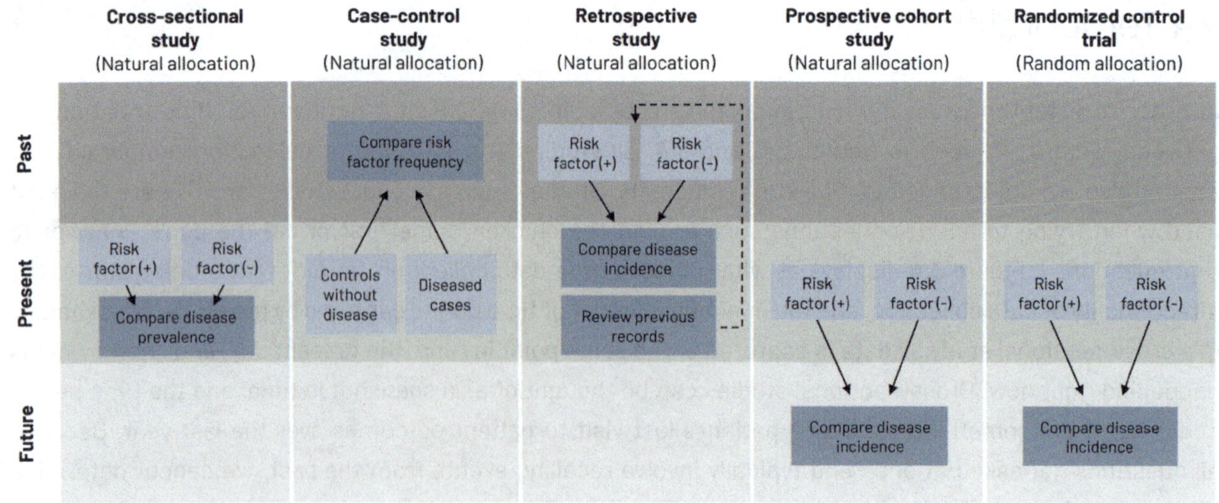

Figure 3.6: Temporality.

3.4 Observational Study Designs

Ecological studies use group summary measures for exposure and outcome rather than measures about individual people. We would use this type of study to compare populations, such as the rate of disease in France compared to the United States or the rate of disease in the United States in 1950 compared to 2000. Because this type of study compares groups, we cannot assume that the results from this study should apply to individuals. It also means that studies we do using data on individuals should not be assumed to apply to groups. If we were to do that, we would be committing the **ecologic fallacy**.

Example: Ecologic fallacy

If we find out that the rate of heat-related illnesses during track and field is high in states in the southern United States, that does not automatically mean that individuals in the southern United States have higher risks of heat-related illness than people living other places. It just means that on a group basis, their rates are higher. If we find out that 80 of 100 individual people with heat illness at a track meet are from the southern United States, it does not mean that 80 percent of all heat-related illnesses occur in the southern United States. If we do make these incorrect assumptions, we have just been guilty of the ecological fallacy. We need to do a better job being correct in our *inferences*, or the meaning we assign to the data that we see. It would be a fallacy to assume that people from the southern United States will experience heat illness based on the presentation of data.

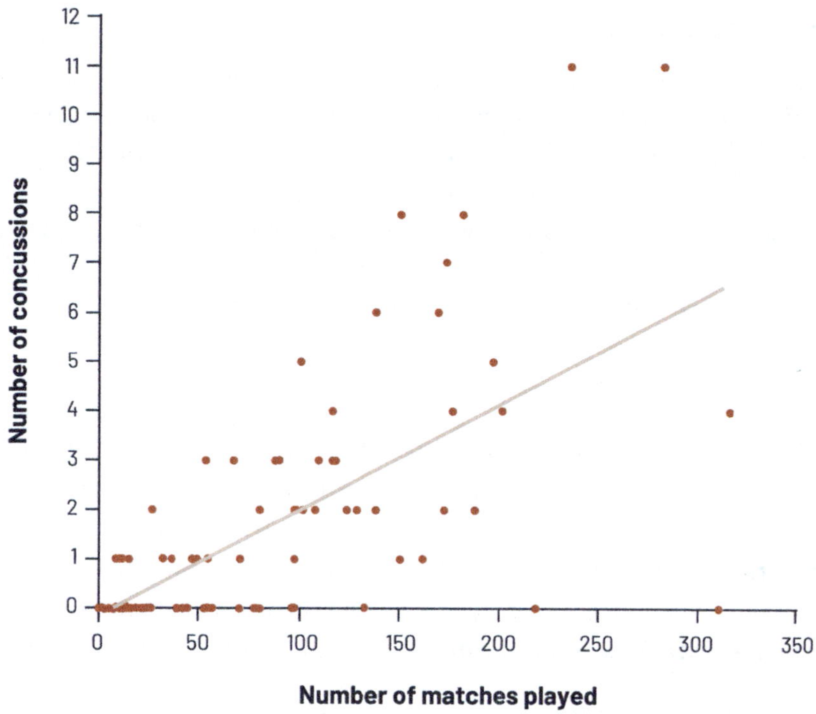

Figure 3.7: Ecological relationship between concussion incidence and matches played.

In this example, we see that there is a positive relationship between the number of Professional Australian Football matches played and the number of concussions that were diagnosed.[2] However, we would not want to assume that every player with more matches will have any concussions. As we can see, at least some players with a high number of matches have no concussions. We also can see that some players with few matches have a higher number of concussions than players with more matches. We can only infer what we see, which is the probability (chance) of an increased risk of concussion with more matches.

In a 2006 TED Talk, statistics expert and physician Hans Rosling provided an excellent example of the importance of ecological studies. You can see it in the first 7 minutes of this video.[3]

Cross-sectional studies measure the prevalence of disease and of exposures (i.e., risk factors) at one point in time. Cross-sectional studies are also known as prevalence studies. When we think about what is being measured in a cross-sectional study, we should think about taking a photo or a *snapshot*: it is a photo of you right now, not what you looked like in the past or what you will look like in the future. We do not know when an exposure happened or when a disease started, we just know they are present *right now*.

Example: Cross-sectional study

During the COVID-19 pandemic, professional athletes in the United States needed to pass cardiac testing in order to return to play after testing positive for COVID-19. Researchers conducted a study to find out the "prevalence of detectable inflammatory heart disease" among athletes in the National Basketball Association, the Women's National Basketball Association, National Hockey League, National Football League, Major League Soccer, and Major League Baseball between May and October 2020.[4] They found that 789 athletes tested positive for COVID-19 and, of those, 30 required further screening.[5] Ultimately, 5 athletes had detectable inflammatory heart disease and were held out of play.

Case-control studies are used to find out *whether a particular exposure could have been the source or cause of a disease*, particularly in urgent health situations. We *start* by identifying who already has the disease (**cases**), then we find a set of people who are like the cases in every respect **except** they do not have disease. These are called **controls**. We ask these cases and controls questions about their past exposures. Because we start with people who are diseased, case-control studies are great when you are interested in studying people who have **rare diseases.** This design is explored more in the next section on Outbreak Investigations.

Cohort studies *start* with a group of individuals based on their *exposure* status. They are used to find out *whether a particular disease comes after a particular exposure or development of a risk factor.* If someone does not have the chance of being exposed, they would not be a good selection for a cohort study. You want everyone to have the potential of getting the outcome because of the exposure. Because of this, cohort studies are great when you're interested in studying people who have **rare exposures**. Once the exposure status is identified, researchers then identify whether or not the subjects have the outcome of interest already. If they do, they would be removed from a prospective study because our goal is to see if the outcome happens *after* the exposure, and if they already have both, how would we know? There are roughly three types of cohort studies: **prospective**, **retrospective**, and **historical**. Every cohort study has *at least two data collection points and they do not overlap*. Prospective means we are setting up the study today and actively following forward into the future. Retrospective means we are setting up the study today but we are looking at information that was previously gathered. So how are retrospective cohort studies different from case-control studies? (See figure 3.6.)

In our next example, we explore how we might approach hospital-acquired infections after anterior cruciate ligament (ACL) reconstruction surgery compared to ACL repair surgery with a cohort study or a case-control study.

Example: Hospital-acquired infections after ACL reconstruction surgery vs ACL repair surgery

Type of question that can be answered with retrospective cohort study: We are interested in identifying whether there are *more* hospital-acquired infections (the outcome) after ACL reconstruction surgery compared to ACL repair surgery (the exposure).

In a retrospective cohort study, we would start by identifying everyone in the population under study (e.g., all patients seen at hospital A) who was eligible for ACL surgery using hospital records. We would select from this population people who had either the ACL reconstruction or ACL repair surgery at Hospital A. We then go through their records to identify what happened to them ***prior*** *to having the surgery and then move forward through their records to see whether they developed a hospital-acquired infection after surgery. Measurement 1: Eligibility for study (exposure status) and determination of whether they already had the outcome* ***before*** *the surgery (which would exclude them). Measurement 2: Determination of whether they had the outcome* ***after*** *the surgery. This provides evidence that the hospital-acquired infection came after the surgery but doesn't rule out that it could have been caused in full or in part by something else postsurgically.*

Type of question that can be answered with case-control study: Hospital A has a number of hospital-acquired infections after surgery. We are interested in identifying whether ACL reconstruction surgery or ACL repair surgery is more common (exposure) in people who have hospital-acquired infections (cases).

In a case-control study, we would start by identifying everyone in the population under study (e.g., all patients seen at hospital A) who had a hospital-acquired infection after surgery (the outcome) using hospital records. We would find patients in Hospital A who did not have the hospital-acquired infection but could have gotten it from surgery (controls). We would then use existing records or talk to patients/providers/environmental services to find out more info about the potential places in the hospital where they could have gotten the infection. This would have helped us identify the type of surgery as a potential exposure. We would compare the cases with the exposure (e.g., ACL reconstruction surgery) to those without the exposure to see if there was a difference in the chance of having a hospital-acquired infection. Whatever exposures have the higher OR would be the ones we'd investigate further as the potential place to intervene. Measurement 1: Eligibility for study, exposure status, disease status. No second measurement.

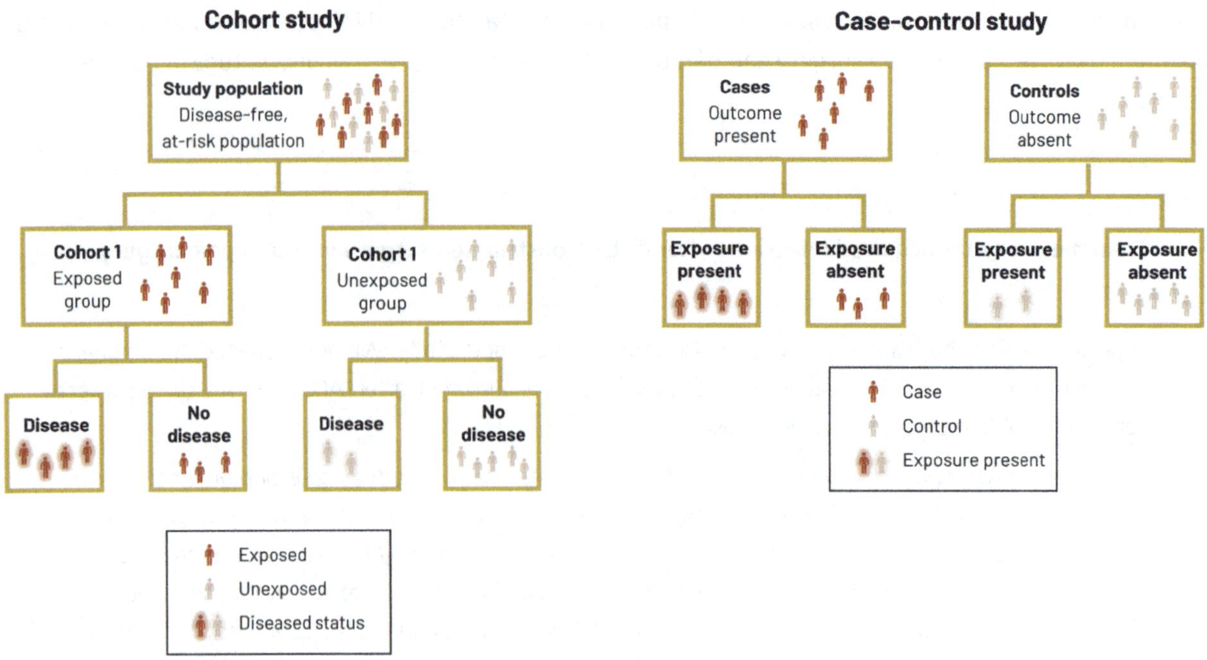

Figure 3.8: Case control versus cohort studies.

3.5 Measures of Association

As noted in section 3.2, we often use a 2x2 table to analyze data from an epidemiological study (figure 3.5). This table is repeated many times in the following text.

	Outcome (+)	**Outcome (-)**	Total outcome
Exposed (+)	**A**	**B**	A + B
Exposed (-)	**C**	**D**	C + D
Total exposed	A + C	B + D	A + B + C + D

Figure 3.9: Example 2x2 table.

***Beware**! While one side of the table above has exposure (or risk factors) and the other side has outcomes (such as disease), everyone does not set their table up the same way (see figure 3.10). Before doing any calculations with data from a 2x2 table, pay attention to how it is set up. All examples in this book use the version showing exposure in rows and outcome in columns.*

	Outcome (-)	**Outcome (+)**
Exposure (-)		
Exposure (+)		

	Exposure (+)	**Exposure (-)**
Outcome (+)		
Outcome (-)		

	Exposure (-)	**Exposure (+)**
Outcome (-)		
Outcome (+)		

Figure 3.10: Example of alternative 2x2 tables.

When we calculate our measures of association, we refer to the needed components by referring to different boxes of our 2x2 table using letters.

- A - Has the outcome and is exposed
- B - Does not have the outcome and is exposed
- C - Has the outcome and is not exposed
- D - Does not have the outcome and is not exposed

Examples of the measures of association are the odds ratio and the relative risk. A measure used in cross-sectional studies is the prevalence rate ratio.

Study design	Measures of disease	Measures of risk	Temporality
Ecological	Prevalence (rough estimate)	Prevalence ratio	Retrospective
Proportional mortality	• Proportional mortality • Standardized mortality	• Proportional mortality ratio • Standardized mortality ratio	Retrospective
Case-crossover	None	Odds ratio	Retrospective
Cross-sectional	• Point prevalence • Period prevalence	• Odds ratio • Prevalence odds ratio • Prevalence ratio • Prevalence difference	Retrospective
Case-control	None	Odds ratio	Retrospective
Retrospective and prospective cohort	• Point prevalence • Period prevalence • Incidence	• Odds ratio • Prevalence odds ratio • Prevalence ratio • Prevalence difference • Attributable risk • Incidence rate ratio • Relative risk • Risk ratio • Hazard ratio	• Retrospective only • Both retrospective and prospective • Prospective only

Figure 3.11: The variety of measures that can be calculated from different study designs.

3.5.1 Odds Ratio

The only measure of association that can be calculated in a case-control study is the **odds ratio** (OR) [the probability of being exposed among cases compared to the probability of being exposed among controls]. This particular odds ratio is referred to as the *odds ratio of exposure*.

$$\text{OR (Exposure)} = \frac{\frac{\frac{A}{A+C}}{\frac{C}{A+C}}}{\frac{\frac{B}{B+D}}{\frac{D}{B+D}}} = \frac{\frac{A}{C}}{\frac{B}{D}} = \frac{AD}{BC}$$

$\frac{A}{C}$ is the ratio of those with the outcome and exposure (A) to those with the outcome but no exposure (C). In other words, what proportion of those that have the outcome have the exposure?

$\frac{B}{D}$ is the ratio of those without the outcome but with the exposure (B) to those without the outcome and with no exposure (D). In other words, what proportion of those that do not have the outcome have the exposure?

The shortcut, $\frac{AD}{BC}$, is called the *cross-product ratio*.

$$\text{OR} = \frac{AD}{BC}$$

The resulting answer is a direct comparison of the ratio of the proportion of those with the exposure who have the outcome to proportion of those with the exposure without the outcome. If this number is *equal* to 1 (roughly, 0.9 to 1.1), there is no difference in the probability of having the exposure between the outcome groups. If this number is greater than 1 (roughly, greater than 1.1), the group with the outcome is more likely to have the exposure than the group without the outcome. If this number is less than 1 (roughly, less than 0.9), the group with the outcome is less likely to have the exposure than the group without the outcome.

OR < 1 (0.9)	**OR = 1** (0.9-1.1)	**OR > 1** (1.1)
Exposure **less likely** in those with outcome compared to those without the outcome	No difference!	Exposure **more likely** in those with outcome compared to those without the outcome

Figure 3.12: Interpreting odds ratios.

Always be specific when drawing comparisons. Just saying, for example, "Cases are 3.2 times more likely to have the exposure" is an incomplete interpretation of the OR. "Cases are 3.2 times more likely to have the exposure compared to controls" is clear about what you are comparing the odds of cases to. This applies to relative risk interpretations as well.

We can also calculate an OR (of exposure or disease) in other study designs, including cross-sectional, cohort, and RCTs. How it gets interpreted in these cases is often different than how we interpret it in a case-control based on the nature of the study and the difference in the full calculation.

3.5.2 Relative Risk

The primary measure of association that is calculated in a cohort study is the **relative risk** (the risk or incidence of the outcome in the exposed compared to the risk or incidence of the outcome in the unexposed).

$\frac{A}{A+B}$ is the incidence (or risk) of disease (A) in the exposed (A+B). $\frac{C}{C+D}$ is the incidence (or risk) of disease (C) in the unexposed (C+D). The relative risk is the ratio of the incidence of disease in the exposed to the incidence of disease in the unexposed. In other words, how is the risk of disease in the exposed different than the risk of disease in the unexposed?

If this number is *equal* to 1 (roughly, 0.9 to 1.1), there is no difference in the risk between exposure groups. If this number is greater than 1 (roughly, greater than 1.1), the group with the exposure is more likely to have the disease than the group without the exposure. If this number is less than 1 (roughly, less than 0.9), the group with the exposure is less likely to have the disease than the group without the exposure.

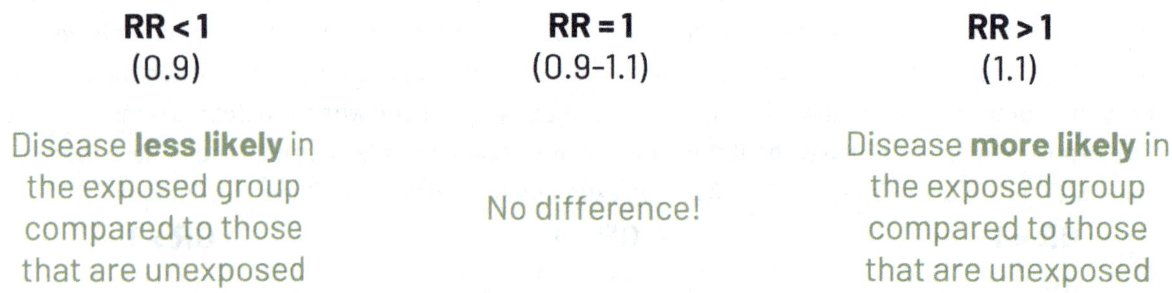

Figure 3.13: Interpreting relative risks.

Calculating the odds ratio in a cohort study means that we are calculating the **odds ratio of disease**. This is calculated differently than the odds ratio of exposure that we calculate in a case-control study (see above). While both formulas result in the cross-product ratio, because they were calculated differently we interpret them differently. Remember that cohort studies are to identify the *risk of disease in the exposed compared to the risk of disease in the unexposed*.

$$\text{OR (Disease)} = \frac{\frac{\frac{A}{A+B}}{\frac{B}{A+B}}}{\frac{\frac{C}{C+D}}{\frac{D}{C+D}}} = \frac{\frac{A}{B}}{\frac{C}{D}} = \frac{AD}{BC}$$

3.5.3 Prevalence Rate Ratio

As noted earlier, prevalence is:

$$\text{Prevalence} = \frac{\text{All cases right now}}{\text{Whole population}}$$

In cross-sectional studies, a common measure of association we calculate is the *prevalence rate ratio*. While the name is a misnomer (prevalence is a proportion, not a rate), it still uses a familiar formula to compare things like the prevalence between either two separate groups (e.g., injury prevalence in Oklahoma compared to injury prevalence in Texas) or the same group at different points in time (e.g., injury prevalence in Virginia in 2015 compared to injury prevalence in Virginia in 2020).

$$\text{Prevalence rate ratio (PRR)} = \frac{\text{Prevalence in group A}}{\text{Prevalence in group B}}$$

$$\text{Prevalence rate ratio (PRR)} = \frac{\frac{A}{A+B}}{\frac{C}{C+D}}$$

3.6 Outbreak Investigations

An **outbreak** is the occurrence of disease in an *area* at a level exceeding the normally *expected number of cases*. An outbreak technically differs from an **epidemic** because an outbreak occurs in a more limited geographic area. Epidemics are declared by country-specific health bodies (e.g., the US Centers for Disease Control and Prevention). A disease is **endemic** if it is occurring at a level expected. It is normally occurring in that place. An epidemic becomes a **pandemic** when the World Health Organization decides it has become one. A pandemic is an epidemic that is spread over multiple countries or continents. Epidemics and pandemics can have variable time patterns, as seen in section 2.4.

One of the most common ways that outbreaks are identified is through clinicians paying attention to changes in what they are treating and who they are treating. Figure 3.14 displays the 11 steps to solving an outbreak.[6]

1. Establish the existence of an outbreak
2. Verify the diagnosis
3. Construct a working case definition
4. Find cases systematically and record information
5. Perform descriptive epidemiology
6. Develop hypotheses
7. Evaluate hypotheses epidemiologically
8. As necessary, reconsider, refine, and re-evaluate hypotheses
9. Compare and reconcile with laboratory and/or environmental studies
10. Implement control and prevention measures
11. Initiate or maintain surveillance findings

These steps often happen simultaneously

Figure 3.14: Steps to solving an outbreak.

Step 1: Establish the existence of an outbreak.

Step 2: Verify the diagnosis.

Before we expend too many resources and too much time, we want to be sure that we are actually observing an outbreak. Things that could look like an outbreak but are not:

- Misdiagnosis/false report:
  - False positive (specificity)
  - Laboratory error
  - Change in case definition
  - Incorrect time or place
  - False report
- Changes in:
  - Awareness
  - Record keeping
  - Observation
  - Population composition

Sometimes we improve our surveillance systems or other tracking methods and pick up more cases because we are doing a better job. This does not mean we actually have more cases, we just are doing a better job at seeing them. Other times, we simply make mistakes in identification that could make it appear like we have more cases. Besides these things, we start calculating our prevalence and incidence, as well as if there are reasonable explanations for changes in these numbers, to determine whether to proceed. We should calculate prevalence if we need to know the total burden of the problem. We should calculate incidence if we are trying to find the risk of developing a disease in a given time. Sometimes we need to do both. The most important part of steps 1 and 2 is that we must verify that the diagnosis we think is the problem is in fact the correct diagnosis. For example, if we think that we are having an outbreak of meningitis A, we should confirm that all of the people who are sick actually have meningitis A.

Our goal is to identify all of the following:

- Individual: Who is affected?
- Place: Where are they affected?
- Time: When did this start or change?
- Connections: What factors are related?

Moving forward in an outbreak investigation is all about what we think, what we know, and what we can prove.

Step 3: Construct a working case definition.

Taking this information, we move into Step 3 and create a working case definition. Many times, this definition stays in flux. Using our case definition, we identify the individual cases, controls, and possible/suspected cases.

Case definitions include a standard set of criteria used to determine if an individual should be classified as a case. Depending on the condition or disease in question, case definitions may already be established. In other situations, this needs to be developed as the investigation progresses. Sometimes the disease or condition in question is required to be reported to the health department or the Centers for Disease Control and Prevention. Nationally notifiable conditions are reported to the National Notifiable Diseases Surveillance System.[7] Each state also has a separate list of notifiable conditions. For example, Virginia's conditions are reported to the Virginia Department of Health and the State Board of Health.[8]

A case definition usually includes both:

- Clinical criteria and/or lab test
- Restrictions by time, place, and/or person

When developing the case definition, we tend to emphasize sensitivity (to identify all possible cases) over specificity (to identify only "true" cases). Part of this is because it is better to err with caution and include too many people than not all cases, especially in the beginning of the investigation. Sensitivity and specificity are discussed in more detail in chapter 4.

Example: Case definition

In figure 3.15, we see the diagnostic criteria for hemophagocytic lymphohistiocytosis (HLH), a rare syndrome of excessive immune response. In order to be considered someone who has HLH, a person must have most but not all diagnostic criteria. However, sometimes not all patients will have all tests that are required to be considered a case. If they meet several criteria, they are instead what is known as a *possible* or *probable* case.

1 **Familial disease/known genetic defect**

2 **Clinical and laboratory criteria (5/8 criteria should be fulfilled)**

- Fever
- Splenomegaly
- Cytopenia ≥2 cell lines
  - Hemoglobin <90 g/l (below 4 weeks of age <120 g/l)
  - Platelets <100 x 10^9/l
  - Neutrophils <1 x 10^9/l
- Hypertriglyceridemia and/or hypofibrinogenemia
  - Fasting triglycerides ≥3 mmol/l
  - Fibrinogen <1.5 g/l
- Ferritin ≥500 μg/l
- Soluble IL-2 receptor 25 ≥2,400 U/ml
- Decreased or absent natural killer cell activity
- Hemophagocytosis in bone marrow, cerebrospinal fluid, or lymph nodes

Supportive evidence is cerebral symptoms with moderate pleocytosis and/or elevated protein, elevated transaminases, bilirubin, lactate dehydrogenase.

Figure 3.15: Example case definition. **[Case: meets all criteria. Possible case: meets several criteria but missing some tests or features.]**

Step 4: Find cases systematically and record information.

Once we have a case definition, we can then work to find all cases (Step 4). We must do this in a systematic fashion and record data on any cases or potential cases we find. We make every effort to find cases that occurred earlier than when we first realized something might be amiss. We use a **line listing** to organize the data about our cases. In figure 3.16, we see an example of a line listing from an anthrax outbreak. Each row corresponds to a different case, and we include all the possible details relevant to the case status and demographic information.

Case no.	Onset date, 2001	Date of anthrax diagnosis by lab testing	State	Age (years)	Sex	Race	Occupation	Case status	Anthrax presentation	Outcome	Diagnostic tests
1	9/22	10/19	NY	31	F	W	*NY Post* employee	Suspect	Cutaneous	Alive	Serum IgG reactive
2	9/25	10/12	NY	38	F	W	NBC anchor assistant	Confirmed	Cutaneous	Alive	Skin biopsy IHC+/ Serum IgG reactive
3	9/26	10/18	NJ	39	M	W	USPS machine mechanic	Suspect	Cutaneous	Alive	Serum IgG reactive

Figure 3.16: *Example* line listing.

Step 5: Perform descriptive epidemiology.

In Step 5, we perform descriptive epidemiology on the data we have gathered from clinical records, questionnaires, interviews, and so on. Just as with several other conditions, if it is a suspected foodborne outbreak, we can use tools from CDC[9] to gather all the pertinent details. We are specifically looking for patterns and associations between risk factors and disease. All the information we will compare is in our line listing. Our measures of association and effect are very useful at this step.

If it is a foodborne outbreak, instead of calculating incidence as we learned before, we usually reframe risk as the **attack rate** (figure 3.17).

$$\text{Attack rate} = \frac{\text{Number ill that ate a food}}{\text{Number that ate a food}} \times 100$$

We can use this to find what percentage of those at risk are actually ill.

	Sick (Outcome)	**Not sick** (Outcome)
Ate salad (Exposure)	48	20
Didn't eat salad (Exposure)	2	100

Figure 3.17: Example attack rate: How big is the difference between groups?

$$\text{Attack rate} = \frac{48}{48+20} \times 100 = 70.6 \text{ percent}$$

We interpret the attack rate as the percentage of those with the exposure that are sick. In the above example, 70.6 percent of those that ate salad are sick. We would compare attack rates to determine which exposures deserve more attention as possible causes.

Step 6: Develop hypotheses.

Step 7: Evaluate hypotheses epidemiologically.

In Steps 6 and 7, we form hypotheses based on our existing data and test them. Among other things, our hypotheses may relate to:

- Cause of the outbreak
- Risk factors for disease
- Risk factors for infection
- Intervention to stop spread: quarantine and vaccinate
- Treatment of affected individuals

Step 8: As necessary, reconsider, refine, and reevaluate hypotheses.

Step 9: Compare and reconcile with laboratory and/or environmental studies.

Step 10: Implement control and prevention measures.

Step 11: Initiate or maintain surveillance findings.

Our final steps of an outbreak investigation are to continue refining our hypotheses, compiling more data to support or refute our hypotheses, controlling the outbreak, and performing surveillance to keep an eye on the problem. Sometimes we find the source of the problem but cannot just "solve" it. The cost of treating the problem, the cost of the intervention to fix the problem, and the existence of other alternatives all play into our decision about what to do. Controlling the problem might include vaccine development and distribution, it might be stopping access to a dangerous substance, or recalling food products.

In the case of some problems, like COVID-19 or sickle cell disease, we initiate and maintain an ongoing systematic data collection system. This is known as **disease surveillance**. The US Centers for Disease Control and Prevention reports on the surveillance of notifiable diseases in both the Morbidity and Mortality Weekly Report[10] (MMWR) and CDC WONDER.[11]

3.7 Measures of Effect

When we are comparing results from our study, we compare the measures that we found. Often, we look at:

A. How big is the difference between groups or individuals with and without a particular risk factor? (Magnitude of effect; ratio, difference)
B. Could the difference we found be just due to chance variation? (Significance of effect; p values)
C. How certain are we of the size of the effect? (Precision of, or uncertainty in, estimate; confidence intervals)

We specifically discuss A in this book. More details on B and C can be found in many books on biostatistics.

We already looked at whether one factor was associated with (or related to) another factor or whether an outcome was associated with an exposure. But in the grand scheme of things, what does that really mean for the population we are focused on?

Measures of effect (how big is the effect of an exposure or risk factor) include the **attributable risk** (attributable fraction) and the **population attributable risk** (population attributable fraction). Sometimes epidemiologists and others will refer to these as more **measures of association** rather than separating them into their own category. Because they are very interrelated, it does not matter whether you refer to them as measures of effect or measures of association but rather when and how to use them. When we're focused on population health, looking at relative differences like the odds ratio or relative risk is extremely useful to decide where we want to make a difference and what factors we should spend our time and energy on. But when we're trying to figure out how to approach the problem at the individual level (for your patient for example), absolute measures can be much more useful.

3.7.1 Attributable Risk

	Outcome (+)	Outcome (-)	Total outcome	Risk
Exposed (+)	A	B	A + B	$\frac{A}{A+B}$
Exposed (-)	C	D	C + D	$\frac{C}{C+D}$
Total exposed	A + C	B + D	A - B + C + D	

Figure 3.18: Using a 2x2 table to calculate attributable risk.

Of everyone that has the exposure, how much of the occurrence of the disease is due to the exposure in question? That's the **attributable risk**. In other words, what's the difference in how much disease we could already expect without the exposure (risk in the unexposed) and how much disease we have if the exposure is present (the risk in the exposed)? This could also be called the **risk difference**. The risk in the unexposed is often referred to as the **baseline risk**.

Example: Attributable risk

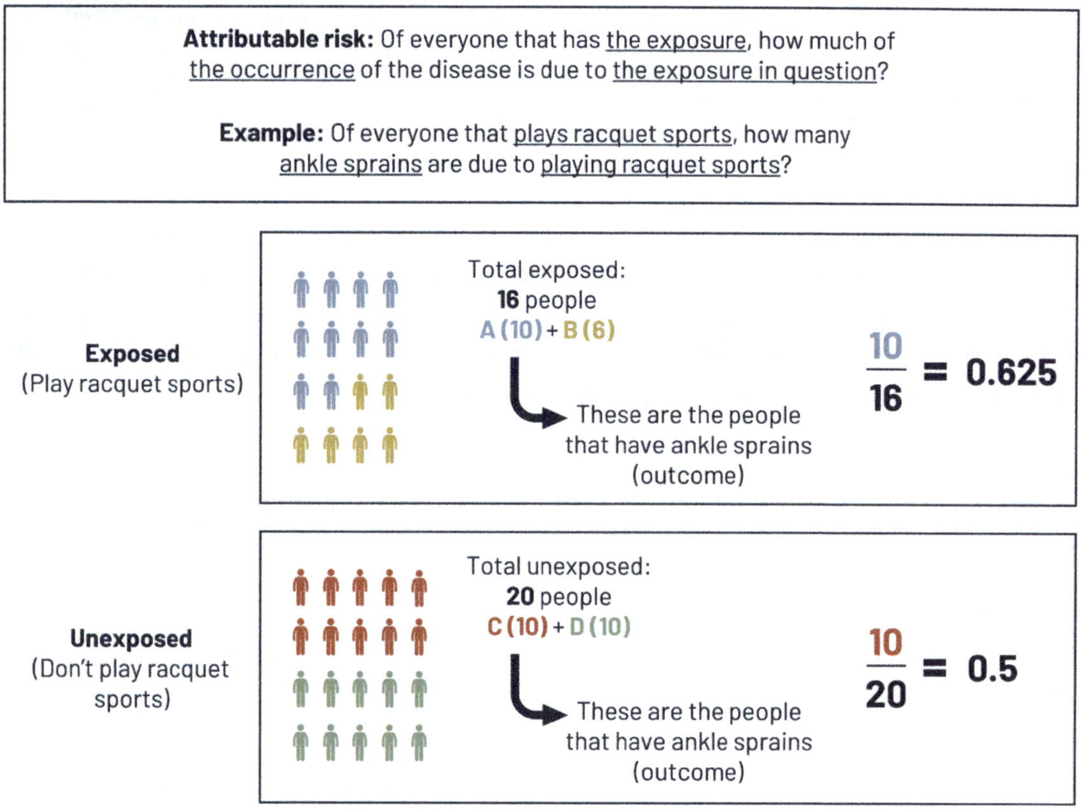

Figure 3.19: Calculating attributable risk.

In our example, the risk of disease in the exposed group is $\frac{10}{16}$ (0.625). The risk of disease in the unexposed group is $\frac{10}{20}$ (0.500). The attributable risk is the difference between these two numbers:

$$AR = 0.625 - 0.500 = 0.125$$

The number we get—0.125—is called an *absolute* number that tells us how different the risk is for the exposed than the risk for the unexposed. For improved understanding, we tend to make it *relative* by turning it into a percentage.

$$\text{AR percent} = \frac{\text{Risk in the exposed - Risk in the unexposed}}{\text{Risk in the exposed}} \times 100$$

$$\text{AR percent} = \frac{0.625-0.500}{0.625} \times 100 = 20 \text{ percent}$$

The AR percent tells us what percent of the risk of disease *in the exposed group* is ***attributable*** to the exposure itself. In this case, 20 percent of the risk of an ankle sprain in those that play racquet sports is due to those people playing racquet sports.

When we use attributable risk to see how well a clinical intervention (e.g., a vaccination) performs, we know that the relative risk correlates to how well the intervention will perform. If the relative risk is < 1 (lower risk of the outcome due to the intervention), then the AR will be negative. This is what happens if the intervention works! If the relative risk is > 1 (higher risk of the outcome due to the intervention), then the AR will be positive. This is what happens when the intervention is not that great.

Further reading

Check out this article on the use of the risk difference and the relative risk when comparing the effectiveness of treatment options.[12]

3.7.2 Measures Especially Important in Clinical Medicine

If we can figure out the attributable risk, we can also identify the **relative risk reduction**, the **absolute risk reduction**, the **number needed to treat**, and the **number needed to harm**.

Measure	Equation	Which way to round
Relative risk reduction (RRR)	$\text{Relative risk reduction (RRR)} = 1 - \text{relative risk}$	-
Absolute risk reduction (ARR)	$\text{Absolute risk reduction } (ARR) = \left\lvert \frac{C}{C+D} - \frac{A}{A+B} \right\rvert$	Neither. Take the absolute value.
Number needed to treat (NNT)	$\text{Number needed to treat (NNT)} = \frac{1}{\text{absolute risk reduction}}$	Up
Number needed to harm (NNH)	$\text{Number needed to harm (NNH)} = \frac{1}{\text{attributable risk}}$	Down

Figure 3.20: Summary of important clinical medicine measures.

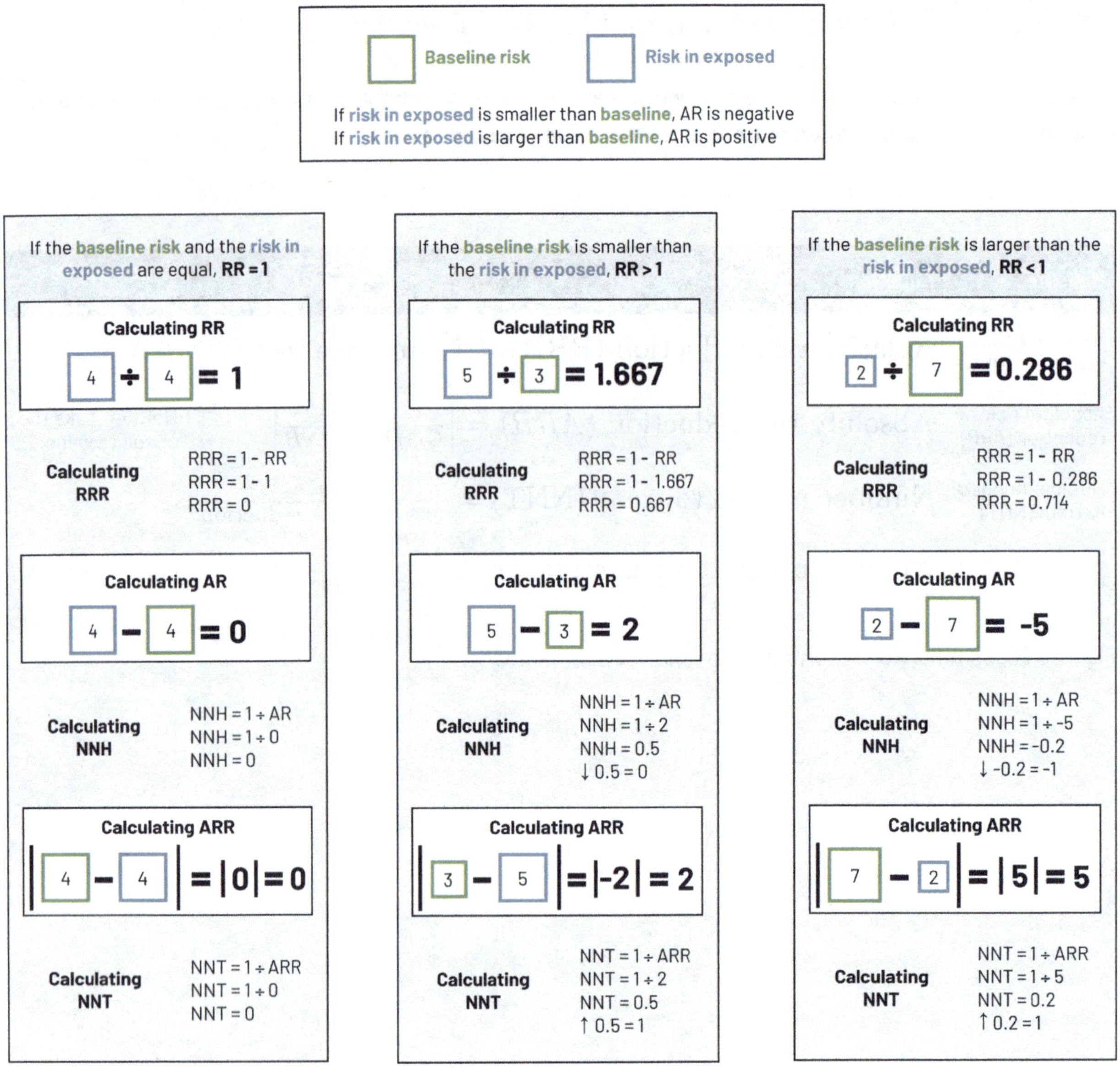

Figure 3.21: Graphical representation of figure 3.20.

The **relative risk reduction**: If there is a reduction in the risk of the outcome when a particular intervention is used, how much of that is due to the intervention compared to the control?

$$\text{Relative risk reduction (RRR)} = 1 \text{ - relative risk}$$

The **absolute risk reduction** (also known as the **risk difference**): While the ARR and the AR can both be referred to as the *risk difference*, there is a distinct difference between the two. AR refers to the difference in risk for the outcome among the exposed due to the exposure itself. The ARR is broader and refers to the difference in risk for the outcome in the group that did not have the intervention and the risk for the outcome in the group that did have the intervention.

$$\text{Absolute risk reduction } (ARR) = \left|\frac{C}{C+D} - \frac{A}{A+B}\right|$$

Note

Remember that the vertical bars mean that we take the absolute value of anything between them. So mathematically, | -3 | is equal to 3. We should remember that the difference was negative, so we can take that into account later.

The **number needed to treat**: How many patients have to be treated in order to make a difference for one patient?

$$\text{Number needed to treat (NNT)} = \frac{1}{\text{absolute risk reduction}}$$

Always round the result of the NNT formula *up*.

The **number needed to harm**: How many patients have to be exposed to a risk factor in order to harm one patient?

$$\text{Number needed to harm (NNH)} = \frac{1}{\text{attributable risk}}$$

Always round the result of the NNH formula *down*.

These four measures (NNH, NNT, ARR, and RRR) are very important in clinical medicine.[13] Figure 3.22 provides an example of how to calculate these statistics.

Example: NNH, NNT, ARR, RRR

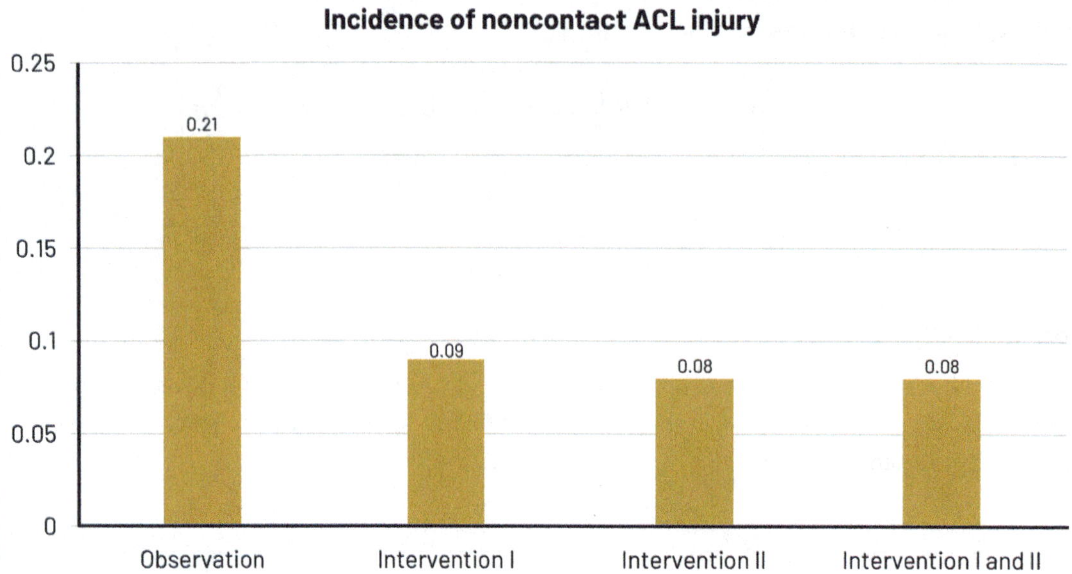

Figure 3.22: EXAMPLE NNH, NNT, ARR, RRR: Noncontact anterior cruciate ligament (ACL) injuries per 1000 athlete-exposures during each period.

Female athletes have a greater risk for ACL injury than male athletes for a variety of reasons. Some 70 percent of ACL injuries in female athletes are due to reasons other than coming in contact with an object or a person. Basketball players are at risk for ACL injury due to the movements they make during play. A study was conducted by Omi et al.[14] to identify the effectiveness of an intervention that aimed to alter risk factors like landing mechanics, muscular strength, postural control, and hip joint control.

The graphic shown (figure 3 from the manuscript[15]) shows the following rates:

- Incidence rate of noncontact ACL injury for 309 athletes who did not receive an intervention (the initial observation period) [Total of 13 injuries]
- Incidence rate for 268 athletes who received Intervention I (players used a ball to simulate basketball rebounding motions and worked to have appropriate knee alignment during landing) [Total of five injuries]
- Incidence rate for 268 athletes who received Intervention II (an upgrade to Intervention I that included [a] application of a flexible band at the thigh level in all jump-landing maneuvers except for contact jump to reduce hip adduction, hip internal rotation, and knee valgus; [b] implementation of hip external rotation strengthening in addition to hip abduction strengthening; and [c] enhancement in quality of balance exercises such as cross-leg hop forward and side hop) [Total of three injuries]

- Combined incidence rate for Interventions I and II

If you need more numbers to follow along, download the manuscript17 from PubMed. Remember that rounding differently and using the rates per 1000 athlete-exposures (aka, person-time) as opposed to incidence per total in the group results in differences in numbers during calculations.

For the purpose of our example, we'll refer only to the Observation, Intervention I, and Intervention II parts of the graphic.

- Risk of noncontact ACL injury during Observation = 0.21
- Risk of noncontact ACL injury during Intervention I = 0.09
- Risk of noncontact ACL injury during Intervention II = 0.08

How much of the risk of noncontact ACL injury during Intervention I is due to participating in Intervention I?

If we are comparing Intervention I to the Observation (which can be considered baseline since no intervention has taken place):

$$\text{Relative risk} = \frac{0.09}{0.21} = 0.43$$

Athletes who participate in Intervention I have 0.43 times the risk of a noncontact ACL injury compared to athletes at baseline. Intervention I seems to reduce the risk of noncontact ACL injury.

$$\text{Attributable risk (risk difference)} = 0.09 - 0.21 = -0.13$$

Our risk difference is negative. The risk of a noncontact ACL injury is reduced by 13 percent in those who participate in Intervention I.

$$\text{Relative Risk Reduction} = 1 - 0.43 = 0.57$$

The intervention reduces the risk of noncontact ACL injuries by 57 percent.

$$\text{Absolute Risk Reduction} = \frac{13}{309} - \frac{5}{286} = 0.04 - 0.02 = 0.025$$

The intervention reduces the risk of noncontact ACL injury 2.5 percent compared to baseline.

$$\text{Number Needed to Treat} = \frac{1}{0.025} = = 40$$

To prevent a noncontact ACL injury in just 1 athlete, 40 athletes must participate in the intervention.

Number Needed to Harm = N/A [There is a positive NNT, so there is no NNH for Intervention I]

If we are comparing Intervention II to the Observation:

$$\text{Relative risk} = \frac{0.08}{0.21} = 0.38$$

Athletes who participate in Intervention II have 0.38 times the risk of a noncontact ACL injury compared to athletes at baseline. Intervention II seems to reduce the risk of noncontact ACL injury.

Attributable risk (risk difference) = 0.08 – 0.21 = -0.14

Our risk difference is negative. The risk of a noncontact ACL injury is reduced by 14 percent in those who participate in Intervention II.

Relative Risk Reduction = 1 – 0.38 = 0.62

The intervention reduces the risk of noncontact ACL injuries by 62 percent.

$$\text{Absolute Risk Reduction} = \frac{13}{309} - \frac{3}{268} = 0.03$$

The intervention reduces the risk of noncontact ACL injury 3 percent compared to baseline.

Number Needed to Treat = 1/0.03 = 34

To prevent a noncontact ACL injury in just 1 athlete, 34 athletes must participate in the intervention.

Number Needed to Harm = N/A [There is a positive NNT, so there is no NNH for Intervention II]

Both the relative risk of noncontact ACL injury after Intervention I and after Intervention II are less than half the risk of noncontact ACL injury when no intervention was used. Intervention II had a slight improvement over Intervention I for how much it reduced the risk of noncontact ACL injury when comparing the absolute risk reductions vs baseline (3 percent vs 2.5 percent).

Attributable risk and its derivatives are important when we are considering a specific population, but often when we develop medications or create other interventions we are considering how much impact they will have on the overall burden of a health problem. Extending our example (figure 3.22), how many noncontact ACL injuries could we have eliminated from the entire population if we eliminated them from women's basketball? The answer to this question is the **population attributable risk**. The population attributable risk is the absolute level of risk of the outcome in the whole population due to the exposure. The difference between this and the attributable risk is that this applies to the risk reduction *even in those that do not have the exposure*. One way to calculate this is:

$$\text{PAR} = \frac{AR}{\frac{\text{Total exposed}}{\text{Total in the population}}}$$

Exposure = Women's basketball **Outcome =** Noncontact ACL injuries

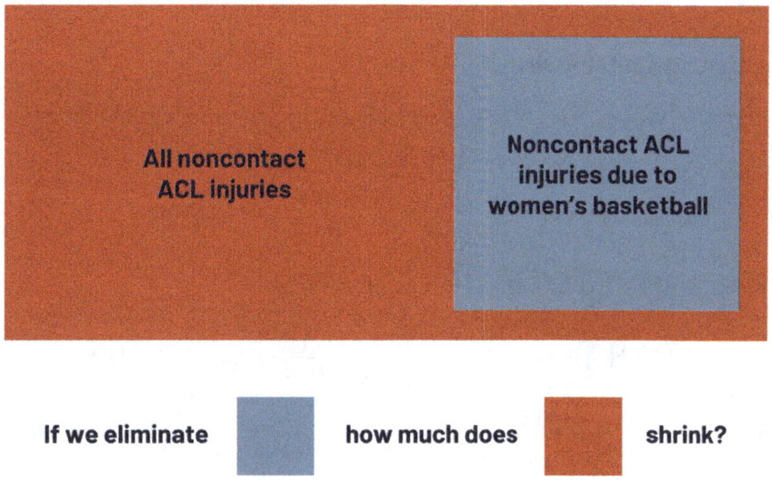

$$\text{PAR} = \frac{\left(\underbrace{\frac{A}{A+B}}_{\text{Risk in exposed}} - \underbrace{\frac{C}{C+D}}_{\text{Risk in unexposed}}\right)}{\left(\text{Number exposed} \div \text{Total population}\right)}$$

Figure 3.23: Calculating the population attributable risk using women's basketball injuries.

Example: Population attributable risk

Say there are 4500 NCAA women's basketball players. Based on our example data for Intervention I:

$$AR = -0.14$$

$$\text{PAR} = \frac{-0.14}{\frac{268}{4500}} = \frac{-0.14}{0.06} = -2.3$$

Just like the AR, it can be easier to understand this as a percentage.

$$\text{PAR percent} = \left\{ \frac{AR}{(A+B)*\left[\frac{A+C}{N}\right]} \right\} * 100$$

$$\text{PAR percent} = \frac{-0.14}{(268)*\left[\frac{309}{4500}\right]} = \frac{-0.14}{(268)*(0.07)} = \frac{-0.14}{18.76} = |-0.007 * 100|$$

$$= 0.75 \text{ percent}$$

By implementing Intervention II among all NCAA women's basketball players, we would reduce the total burden of noncontact ACL injuries in this population by less than 1 percent. This intervention may work well on an individual level but not as a population level intervention for noncontact ACL injuries.

Further reading

Want to dive deeper into how the ARR and the RRR should (and shouldn't) be used in real life?

Here's a great explanation related to how not to confuse the public with the COVID-19 vaccination.[16]

Here's a helpful video on how to calculate the NNT.[17]

Interested in why you need the RR to calculate the AR?[18]

Here's an article on how to use risk difference, risk ratio, and odds ratio in clinical medicine.[19]

3.8 Reporting Results of Epidemiologic and Clinical Studies

There are various standards for the reporting of study results and methods. Figure 3.24 provides an example list of different standards. You can find additional standards for various disciplines and different types of studies at the EQUATOR network website.[20]

Standard name	Acronym	Website
Consolidated standards of reporting trials	CONSORT	www.consort-statement.org
Strengthening the reporting of observational studies in epidemiology	STROBE	www.strobe-statement.org
Standards for reporting studies of diagnostic accuracy	STARD	http://dx.doi.org/10.1136/bmjopen-2016-012799
Quality assessment of diagnostic accuracy studies	QUADAS	www.bris.ac.uk/quadas
Preferred reporting items for systematic reviews and meta-analyses	PRISMA	www.prisma-statement.org
Consolidated criteria for reporting qualitative research	COREQ	https://doi.org/10.1093/intqhc/mzm042
Statistical analyses and methods in the published literature	SAMPL	https://doi.org/10.1016/j.ijnurstu.2014.09.006
Consensus-based clinical case reporting guideline development	CARE	www.care-statement.org
Standards for quality improvement reporting excellence	SQUIRE	www.squire-statement.org
Consolidated health economic evaluation reporting standards	CHEERS	https://doi.org/10.1136/bmj.f1049
Enhancing transparency in reporting the synthesis of qualitative research	ENTREQ	https://doi.org/10.1186/1471-2288-12-181

Figure 3.24: Standards for study design and reporting.

In addition to reporting study results, it is also normal and helpful to report on how studies were designed and implemented. This reporting of methods helps others better understand all the work that goes into obtaining results as well as potential roadblocks to watch out for when designing a similar study to expand what is known about a topic. The CARE Consortium published a journal article in 2017 about how they built a national study of concussion in service academy students and collegiate athletes with the Department of Defense.[21]

Figure Descriptions

Figure 3.1: Flow chart. Following pathway to left: Controlled assignment of subjects to study conditions arrow to randomized (clinical trials) or non-randomized/ quasi-experimental (community trials). Clinical trials and community trials are types of experimental studies. Following pathway to right: Uncontrolled/not randomized assignment of subjects to study conditions, arrow to sampling with regard to exposure, characteristic, or cause (prospective studies). Sampling with regard to disease or effect, arrow to time of exposure/characteristic. Exposure or characteristic at time of study (cross-sectional studies). History of exposure or characteristic prior to time of study (retrospective studies). Prospective studies, retrospective studies, and cross-sectional studies are types of observational studies. Return to figure 3.1.

Figure 3.5: Headers on top of table are outcome (+) and outcome (-). Headers to left of the table are exposed (+) and exposed (-). If outcome (+) and exposed (+), A. If outcome (-) and exposed (+), B. If outcome (+) and exposed (-), C. If outcome (-) and exposed (-), D. Reading left to right in the table: A, B, C, D. Outside of the table are calculations for finding total exposed and total outcome. Below the table left to right: total exposed, A+C, B+D, A+B+C+D. Right of the table top to bottom: total outcome, A+B, C+D, A+B+C+D. Total population represented by A+B+C+D in bottom right corner. Return to figure 3.5.

Figure 3.6: Cross-sectional study (natural allocation): in the present, risk factor (+) and risk factor (-) point to compare disease prevalence. Case-control study (natural allocation): in the present, controls without disease and diseased cases both point to past box stating compare risk factor frequency. Retrospective study (natural allocation): in the past, risk factor (+) and risk factor (-) point to present box stating compare disease incidence; another box in present time states review previous records with a dotted arrow pointing back to the past risk factors. Prospective cohort study (natural allocation): in the present, risk factor (+) and risk factor (-) point to future box stating compare disease incidence. Randomized control trial (random allocation): in the present, risk factor (+) and risk factor (-) point to future box stating compare disease incidence. Return to figure 3.6.

Figure 3.7: X-axis displays number of matches played (ranging from 0 to 350). Y-axis displays number of concussions (ranging from 0 to 12). Roughly 50 data points on the graph with a regression line indicating the average. As number of matches played increases, the number of concussions increases. Return to figure 3.7.

Figure 3.8: Cohort study: study population is disease-free and at-risk. Half of the study population is labeled cohort 1 (exposed group), the other half is labeled cohort 2 (unexposed group). Of the cohort 1 group, there are some with disease and some with no disease. Of the cohort 2 group, there are some with disease and some with no disease. Diseased status in two cohorts is identified. Case control study: there are separate groups based on outcome status. First group: cases (outcome present). Second group: controls (outcome absent). Each of these groups have subgroups where there is either a present exposure or an absent exposure. Return to figure 3.8.

Figure 3.9: Headers on top of table are outcome (+) and outcome (-). Headers to left of the table are exposed (+) and exposed (-). If outcome (+) and exposed (+), A. If outcome (-) and exposed (+), B. If outcome (+) and exposed (-), C. If outcome (-) and exposed (-), D. Reading left to right in the table: A, B, C, D. Outside of the table are calculations for finding total exposed and total outcome. Below the table left to right: total exposed, A+C, B+D, A+B+C+D. Right of the table top to bottom: total outcome, A+B, C+D, A+B+C+D. Total population represented by A+B+C+D in bottom right corner. Return to figure 3.9.

Figure 3.10: Three separate 2x2 tables. First: Outcome (-) and outcome (+) are above the table and exposure (-) and exposure (+) are left of the table. Second: exposure (+) and exposure (-) are above the table and outcome (+) and outcome (-) are left of the table. Third: exposure (-) and exposure (+) are above the table and outcome (-) and outcome (+) are left of the table. Return to figure 3.10.

Figure 3.12: OR < 1 (e.g., 0.9): exposure less likely in those with outcome compared to those without the outcome. OR = 1: no difference. OR > 1 (e.g., 1.1): exposure more likely in those with outcome compared to those without the outcome. Return to figure 3.12.

Figure 3.13: RR < 1 (e.g., 0.9): disease less likely in the exposed group compared to those that are unexposed. RR = 1: no difference. RR > 1 (e.g., 1.1): disease more likely in the exposed group compared to those that are unexposed. Return to figure 3.13.

Figure 3.14: 1: Establish the existence of an outbreak. 2: Verify the diagnosis. 3: Construct a working case definition. 4: Find cases systematically and record information. 5: Perform descriptive epidemiology. 6: Develop hypotheses. 7: Evaluate hypotheses epidemiologically. 8: As necessary, reconsider, refine, and re-evaluate hypotheses. 9: Compare and reconcile with laboratory and/or environmental studies. 10: Implement control and prevention measures. 11: Initiate or maintain surveillance findings. Steps 8-11 often happen simultaneously. Return to figure 3.14.

Figure 3.15: 1: familial disease/known genetic defect. 2: clinical and laboratory criteria (5/8 criteria should be fulfilled). Criteria: fever, splenomegaly, cytopenia greater than or equal to 2 cell lines (hemoglobin less than 90 g/l or less than 120 g/l if below 4 weeks of age, platelets less than 100 x 10^9/l, neutrophils less than 1 x 10^9/l), hypertriglyceridemia and/or hypofibrinogenemia (fasting triglycerides greater than or equal to 3 mmol/l, fibrinogen less than 1.5 g/l), ferritin greater than or equal to 500 mu g/l, soluble IL-2 receptor 25 greater than or equal to 2400 U/ml, decreased or absent natural killer cell activity, hemophagocytosis in bone marrow, cerebrospinal fluid, or lymph nodes. Supportive evidence is cerebral symptoms with moderate pleocytosis and/or elevated protein, elevated transaminases, bilirubin, lactate dehydrogenase. Return to figure 3.15.

Figure 3.17: 2x2 table. Above table labels: sick (outcome) and not sick (outcome). Left table labels: ate salad (exposure) and didn't eat salad (exposure). A: 48 (sick and ate salad). B: 20 (not sick and ate salad). C: 2 (sick and didn't eat salad). D: 100 (not sick and didn't eat salad). Return to figure 3.17.

Figure 3.18: Above the table is outcome (+) and outcome (-). Left of the table is exposed (+) and exposed (-). If outcome (+) and exposed (+), A. If outcome (-) and exposed (+), B. If outcome (+) and exposed (-), C. If outcome (-) and exposed (-), D. Reading left to right in the table: A, B, C, D. Outside of the table are calculations for finding total exposed and total outcome. Below the table left to right: total exposed, A+C, B+D, A+B+C+D. Right of the table top to bottom: total outcome, A+B, C+D, A+B+C+D. Additional rightmost column: risk. A/(A+B) and C/(C+D). Return to figure 3.18.

Figure 3.19: Attributable risk: Of everyone that has the exposure, how much of the occurrence of the disease is due to the exposure in question? Example: Of everyone that plays racquet sports, how many ankle sprains are due to playing racquet sports? Example follows. Total exposed (play racquet sports): 16 people (A=10 and B=6). A represents people that have ankle sprains (outcome). A (10) divided by total exposed (16) equals 0.625. Total unexposed (don't play racquet sports): 20 people (C=10 and D=10). C represents people that have ankle sprains (outcome). C (10) divided by total unexposed (20) equals 0.5. Return to figure 3.19.

Figure 3.21: Three boxed columns with steps for calculations of relative risk reduction, number needed to treat, and number needed to harm based on relative risk. If risk in exposed is smaller than baseline, AR is negative. If risk in exposed is larger than baseline, AR is positive. Left column: When relative risk is equal to one, the baseline risk and risk in exposed are equal. Calculating RR: 4 (risk in exposed) divided by 4 (baseline risk) equals an RR of 1. Calculating AR: 4 (risk in exposed) minus by 4 (baseline risk) equals an AR of 0. Calculating ARR: absolute value of 4 (baseline risk) minus 4 (risk in exposed) equals an ARR of 0. Middle column: When relative risk is greater than one, the baseline risk is smaller than the risk in exposed. Calculating RR: 5 (risk in exposed) divided by 3 (baseline risk) equals an RR of 1.667. Calculating AR: 5 (risk in exposed) minus 3 (baseline risk) equals an AR of 2. Calculating ARR: absolute value of 3 (baseline risk) minus 5 (risk in exposed) equals an ARR of 2. Right column: When relative risk is less than one, the baseline risk is larger than the exposed. Calculating RR: 2 (risk in exposed) divided by 7 (baseline risk) equals an RR of 0.286. Calculating AR: 2 (risk in exposed) minus 7 (baseline risk) equals an AR of -5. Calculating ARR: absolute value of 7 (baseline risk) minus 2 (risk in exposed) equals an ARR of 5. Return to figure 3.21.

Figure 3.22: Bar chart showing incidence of noncontact ACL injury. Incidence on x-axis and rates on y-axis. Observation: 0.21. Intervention one: 0.09. Intervention two: 0.08. Intervention one and two: 0.08. Return to figure 3.22.

Figure 3.23: Exposure = women's basketball. Outcome = Noncontact ACL injuries. Noncontact ACL injuries due to women's basketball is a small subset of all noncontact ACL injuries. If we eliminate the small subset, how much does the all noncontact ACL injuries category shrink? Population attributable risk (PAR) equals (risk in exposed minus risk in unexposed) divided by (number exposed divided by total population). Risk in exposed = A divided by (A+B). Risk in unexposed = C divided by (C+D). Return to figure 3.23.

Figure References

Figure 3.1: Overview of study designs. Kindred Grey. 2022. Adapted under fair use from Lilienfeld AM. Advances in quantitative methods in epidemiology. *Public Health Rep.* 1980;95(5):462–469.

Figure 3.2: Bhopal RS. The concept of risk and fundamental measures of disease frequency: Incidence and prevalence. In: Bhopal, RS. Concepts of epidemiology: Integrating the ideas, theories, principles and methods of epidemiology. Oxford University Press; 2008:201–234.

Figure 3.3: Epidemiological study designs. Adapted under fair use from USMLE First Aid, Step 1.

Figure 3.4: Community trials and clinical trials. Adapted under fair use from USMLE First Aid, Step 1.

Figure 3.5: Example 2x2 table. Kindred Grey. 2022. CC BY 4.0.

Figure 3.6: Temporality. Kindred Grey. 2022. CC BY 4.0.

Figure 3.7: Ecological relationship between concussion incidence and matches played. Kindred Grey. 2022. CC BY 4.0. Data from Gibbs N, Watsford M. Concussion incidence and recurrence in professional Australian football match-play: A 14-year analysis. *J Sports Med* (Hindawi Publ Corp). 2017;2017:2831751. DOI:10.1155/2017/2831751

Figure 3.8: Case control versus cohort studies. Kindred Grey. 2022. Includes person by Gan Khoon Lay from Noun Project (Noun Project License). Adapted under fair use from Song JW, Chung KC. Observational studies: Cohort and case-control studies. *Plast Reconstr Surg.* 2010;126(6):2234–2242. DOI:10.1097/PRS.0b013e3181f44abc

Figure 3.9: Example 2x2 table. Kindred Grey. 2022. CC BY 4.0.

Figure 3.10: Example of alternative 2x2 tables. Kindred Grey. 2022. CC BY 4.0.

Figure 3.11: The variety of measures that can be calculated from different study designs. Thiese MS. Observational and interventional study design types: An overview. Biochem Med (Zagreb). 2014;24(2):199–210. DOI:10.11613/BM.2014.022 (CC BY-NC-ND 3.0)

Figure 3.12: Interpreting odds ratios. Kindred Grey. 2022. CC BY 4.0.

Figure 3.13: Interpreting relative risks. Kindred Grey. 2022. CC BY 4.0.

Figure 3.14: Steps to solving an outbreak. Kindred Grey. 2022. CC BY 4.0. Adapted from CDC. Public Domain.

Figure 3.15: Example case definition. Kindred Grey. 2022. Adapted under fair use from Janka GE. Familial and acquired hemophagocytic lymphohistiocytosis. *Annu Rev Med.* 2012;63:233–246. DOI:10.1146/annurev-med-041610-134208 and Henter J-I, Horne A, Aricó M, et al. HLH-2004: Diagnostic and therapeutic guidelines for hemophagocytic lymphohistiocytosis. *Pediatr Blood Cancer.* 2007;48(2):124–131.

Figure 3.16: Example line listing. Data from table 6.5 of Lesson 6: Investigating an outbreak, from CDC. Public domain.

Figure 3.17: Example attack rate. Kindred Grey. 2022. CC BY 4.0.

Figure 3.18: Using a 2x2 table to calculate attributable risk. Kindred Grey. 2022. CC BY 4.0.

Figure 3.19: Calculating attributable risk. Kindred Grey. 2022. CC BY 4.0.

Figure 3.21: Graphical representation of figure 3.20. Kindred Grey. 2022. CC BY 4.0.

Figure 3.22: EXAMPLE NNH, NNT, ARR, RRR. Kindred Grey. 2022. CC BY 4.0. Data from Omi Y, Sugimoto D, Kuriyama S, et al. Effect of hip-focused injury prevention training for anterior cruciate ligament injury reduction in female basketball players: A 12-year prospective intervention study. *Am J Sports Med.* 2018;46(4):852–861. DOI:10.1177/0363546517749474

Figure 3.23: Calculating the population attributable risk using women's basketball injuries. Kindred Grey. 2022. CC BY 4.0.

Figure 3.24: Standards for study design and reporting. Adapted under fair use from Thiese MS. Observational and interventional study design types: An overview. *Biochem Med* (Zagreb). 2014;24(2):199–210. DOI:10.11613/BM.2014.022 (CC BY-NC-ND 3.0)

Notes

1. Which Came First—The Chicken or the Egg? https://www.youtube.com/watch?v=1a8pl65emDE. AsapSCIENCE via YouTube; 2013.
2. Gibbs N, Watsford M. Concussion incidence and recurrence in professional Australian football match-play: A 14-year analysis. *J Sports Med* (Hindawi Publ Corp). 2017;2017:2831751.
3. Rosling H. The best stats you've ever seen. https://www.youtube.com/watch?v=hVimVzgtD6w. TED via YouTube; 2006.
4. Martinez MW, Tucker AM, Bloom OJ, et al. Prevalence of inflammatory heart disease among professional athletes with prior COVID-19 infection who received systematic return-to-play cardiac screening. *JAMA Cardiol.* 2021;6(7):745–752.
5. Martinez MW, Tucker AM, Bloom OJ, et al. Prevalence of inflammatory heart disease among professional athletes with prior COVID-19 infection who received systematic return-to-play cardiac screening. *JAMA Cardiol.* 2021;6(7):745–752.
6. Centers for Disease Control and Prevention. Investigating an outbreak. In: *Principles of epidemiology.* 3rd ed: U.S. Department of Health and Human Services; 2006:6-1–6-78.
7. Centers for Disease Control and Prevention. Surveillance case definitions for current and historical conditions. https://ndc.services.cdc.gov/. Updated 2023. Accessed September 15, 2023.
8. Virginia Department of Health. Rules and regulations of the Board of Health, Commonwealth of Virginia. https://www.vdh.virginia.gov/surveillance-and-investigation/. Published 2021. Accessed 2021.
9. Centers for Disease Control and Prevention. Investigating outbreaks: Using data to link foodborne disease outbreaks to a contaminated source. https://www.cdc.gov/foodsafety/outbreaks/basics/data-types-collected.html?CDC_AA_refVal=https%3A%2F%2Fwww.cdc.gov%2Ffoodsafety%2Foutbreaks%2Finvestigating-outbreaks%2Findex.html. Published 2016. Accessed 2021.
10. Centers for Disease Control and Prevention. Morbidity and mortality weekly report. https://www.cdc.gov/mmwr/index.html. Published 2022. Accessed 2022.
11. Centers for Disease Control and Prevention. CDC WONDER. http://wonder.cdc.gov. Reviewed 2023. Accessed 15 September 2023.
12. Newcombe RG, Bender R. Implementing GRADE: Calculating the risk difference from the baseline risk and the relative risk. *Evid Based Med.* 2014;19(1):6–8.
13. Irwig L, Irwig J, Trevena L, Sweet M. Relative risk, relative and absolute risk reduction, number needed to treat and confidence intervals. In: *Smart Health Choices: Making Sense of Health Advice.*Hammersmith Press; 2008.
14. Omi Y, Sugimoto D, Kuriyama S, et al. Effect of hip-focused injury prevention training for anterior cruciate ligament injury reduction in female basketball players: A 12-year prospective intervention study. *Am J Sports Med.* 2018;46(4):852–861.
15. Omi Y, Sugimoto D, Kuriyama S, et al. Effect of hip-focused injury prevention training for anterior cruciate ligament injury reduction in female basketball players: A 12-year prospective intervention study. *Am J Sports Med.* 2018;46(4):852–861.
16. Reuters Fact Check. Fact Check: Why relative risk reduction, not absolute risk reduction, is most often used in calculating vaccine efficacy. 2023. https://www.reuters.com/article/factcheck-thelancet-riskreduction/fact-check-why-relative-risk-reduction-not-absolute-risk-reduction-is-most-often-used-in-calculating-vaccine-efficacy-idUSL2N2NK1XA. Accessed 15 September 2023.

17. The NNT Group. theNNT, explained. https://www.thennt.com/thennt-explained/. Accessed 15 September 2023.

18. Noordzij M, van Diepen M, Caskey FC, Jager KJ. Relative risk versus absolute risk: One cannot be interpreted without the other. *Nephrol Dial Transplant*. 2017;32(suppl 2):ii13–ii18.

19. Kim HY. Statistical notes for clinical researchers: Risk difference, risk ratio, and odds ratio. *Restor Dent Endod.* 2017;42(1):72–76.

20. EQUATOR network. Enhancing the QUAlity and Transparency Of health Research. https://www.equator-network.org/. Published 2023. Accessed 15 September 2023.

21. Broglio SP, McCrea M, McAllister T, et al. A national study on the effects of concussion in collegiate athletes and US Military Service Academy members: The NCAA-DoD Concussion Assessment, Research and Education (CARE) consortium structure and methods. *N Zeal J Sports Med*. 2017;47(7):1437–1451.

4. DIAGNOSTICS AND SCREENING

Diagnostic and screening tests are **primary** and **secondary prevention** tools (see section 1.1).

What do we use them for?

- Determine whether a patient is likely to have a disease or condition
  - Diseased vs nondiseased
  - Positive vs negative
  - High vs low risk
  - Exposed vs unexposed
- Describe the burden of the disease or condition in the population (prevalence)

In clinical medicine, diagnostic and screening tests help us answer three questions:

- How do we treat individual patients?
- How does the test we use in our study affect the results of the study?
- In the study we're reviewing, did false positives and false negatives bias the results?

One possible problem with diagnostic and screening tests is that they could be incorrect or give false results. Errors can result in patients being treated when they do not need it or not getting treatment when they do. It also can result in decisions that are not reversible (e.g., selective abortion for a birth defect, suicide for a positive HIV test) and may not be acceptable to the population being served.

4.1 Screening Tests

Screening for disease is the presumptive identification of unrecognized disease or defects by the application of tests, examinations, or other procedures that can be applied rapidly. Positive screening results are followed by diagnostic tests to confirm actual disease. For example, if a newborn tests positive during phenylketonuria (PKU) screening at birth, the phenylalanine loading test is used next to confirm the presence of PKU. Common screening tests include the pap smear, mammogram, blood pressure screening, cholesterol testing, vision tests, and urinalysis. When we conduct screening for disease, there are three very important considerations we should make: the social, scientific, and ethical impacts.

Social

- The health problem should be important for the individual and the community.
- Diagnostic follow-up and intervention should be available to all who require them.
- There should be a favorable cost-benefit ratio.
- Public acceptance must be high.

Scientific

- The natural history of the condition should be adequately understood. This knowledge permits identification of early stages of disease and appropriate biologic markers of progression.
- A knowledge base exists for the efficacy of prevention and the occurrence of side effects.
- Prevalence of the disease or condition is high.

Ethical

- The program can alter the natural history of the condition in a significant proportion of those screened.
    - Always ask yourself if you can do anything about changing the course of disease. If not, there is a potential that the screening does more harm than good.
- There should be suitable and acceptable tests for screening and diagnosis of the condition as well as acceptable, effective methods of prevention.

Example: Screening

An example screening program: ECG for athletes to detect heart issues prior to participation[1] during a preparticipation screening.

4.2 Characteristics of a Good Screening Test

A screening test should be

- Simple—easy to learn and perform.
- Rapid—quick to administer; results available rapidly.
- Inexpensive—good cost-benefit ratio.
- Safe—no harm to participants.
- Acceptable—to target group.

A test may not meet all five criteria, but this should be a goal.

Example: ECG screening

- Simple[2]: Programs exist to teach someone how to be an ECG technician, and skills are also included in clinical training for doctors and nurses. All cardiologists can perform this test.
- Rapid[3]: Takes less than 10 minutes, including the time to attach and detach electrodes from the body. Results are often available within 24 hours.
- Inexpensive: Good cost-benefit ratio for people with greater than low risk for heart issues. Poor cost-benefit ratio for people with low risk for heart issues. More data is needed[4] because the costs depend on insurance but are often less than $300.
- Safe: Risks[5] are minimal and rare.
- Acceptable: Noninvasiveness helps to make the screening acceptable.

4.3 Validity and Reliability

When it comes to screening tests or measurements, we are concerned with **validity** and **reliability**. **Internal validity** is **accuracy**. It describes the ability of a measuring instrument to give a true measure. Internal validity can be evaluated only if an accepted and independent method for confirming the test measurement exists. This accepted and independent method is known as a **gold standard**. **Reliability** is **precision**. It describes the ability of a measuring instrument to give consistent results on repeated trials. When we are measuring the reliability over these **repeated measures**, we are looking for the degree of consistency among repeated measurements of the same individual on more than one occasion.

In figure 4.1, we see information about **precision** (reliability) and **accuracy** (validity). Under the column *visual representation*, we see four dartboard targets. Our first row, **Precision**, contains two targets. In each of these, the darts have been thrown in such a way that they are clustered together. These were hit in the same place over and over—they were thrown *precisely*. In the second row, **Accuracy**, you see two additional targets. In the first, the darts were not only thrown precisely but they were also thrown accurately at the bull's-eye. This is a visual representation of what we would like our research to be: precise and accurate. The last target shows us an example of throwing darts that neither land in the sample place (not precise) nor land at the bull's-eye (not accurate). This is a visual representation of exactly what we do not want to happen in research.

	Mnemonic device	What it is	Things to remember	Visual representation
Precision	Precision = Reliability, Reproducibility	• The consistency and reproducibility of a test • The absence of random variation in a test	• Random error ↓ precision in a test • ↑ precision →↓ standard deviation • ↑ precision →↑ statistical power (1-β)	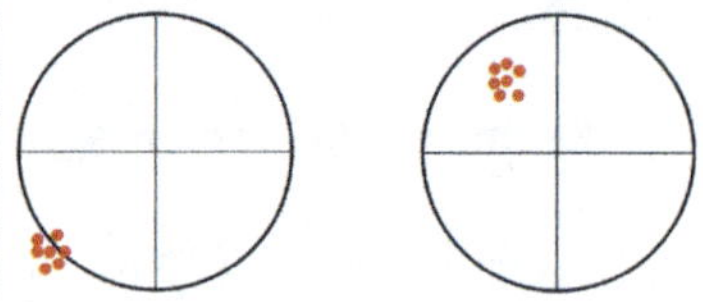
Accuracy	Accuracy = Validity	• The closeness of test results to the true values • The absence of systematic error in a test	Systematic error ↓ accuracy in a test	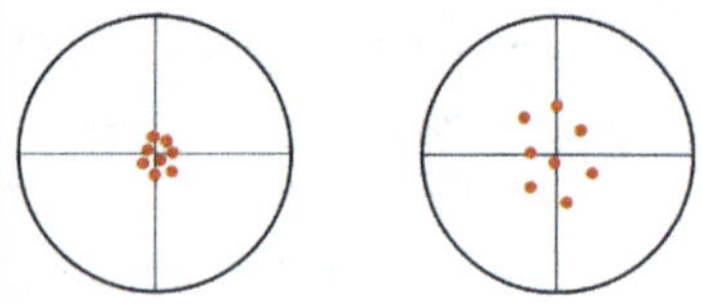

Figure 4.1: Precision and accuracy.

What are some of the things that cause a measure to not be reliable or not be valid?

Measurement bias is when we have constant errors that are introduced by a faulty measuring device. This tends to reduce the reliability of measurements. An example of this is a miscalibrated blood pressure manometer.

The **halo effect** is the influence upon an observation of the observer's perception of the characteristics of the individual observed. This includes the influence of the observer's recollection or knowledge of findings on a previous occasion. An example of this is when a health provider tends to rate a patient's sexual behavior use in a particular manner based on the provider's opinion about the patient's characteristics without obtaining specific information concerning current or past sexual behavior.

Social desirability is when a respondent answers questions in a manner that agrees with socially desirable norms. An example would be when teenage boys respond to a screening interview about sexual behavior by exaggerating their frequency of sexual activities because that might be perceived as socially desirable or cool among their peer groups.

4.4 Measuring Validity and Reliability

When we want to measure the validity of a measuring tool (including screening tests), we use four different measures: **sensitivity**, **specificity**, **positive predictive value**, and **negative predictive value**. It is helpful to use a table when calculating these measures. This table looks similar to the 2×2 table in chapter 3. In figures 4.2 and 4.3, the columns represent the results that the gold standard provides, and the rows represent the results that the new (or comparison) test provides. The table itself helps us calculate how well the test works. If a person is diseased (figure 4.4), our goal is for the test to correctly tell us this. The better the test does, the higher our **sensitivity** (defined below). The better the test is, the more certain we are that if someone tests negative they do not have the disease, so we say that high sensitivity helps us rule out disease. We simultaneously hope for the test to correctly tell us someone does not have the disease. The better the test does at this, we say the higher the **specificity**. The higher the specificity, the more we feel we can rule in disease if someone tests positive. We must balance the two items to make the best test possible, but as noted below, sometimes we sacrifice one to improve the other.

		Condition according to gold standard			
		Present	Absent	Total	
Test result	Positive	A	B	A + B	**Predictive value (+)** $\frac{A}{A+B}$
	Negative	C	D	C + D	**Predictive value (-)** $\frac{D}{C+D}$
	Total	A + C	B + D	Grand total A + B + C + D	
		Sensitivity $\frac{A}{A+C}$	**Specificity** $\frac{D}{B+D}$		

Figure 4.2: The fourfold (2×2) table.

	Disease (+)	Disease (-)	
Test (+)	True positive	False positive	Predictive value (+) $\frac{TP}{TP+FP}$
Test (-)	False negative	True negative	Predictive value (-) $\frac{TN}{TN+FN}$
	Sensitivity $\frac{TP}{TP+FN}$	Specificity $\frac{TN}{TN+FP}$	**Prevalence** $\frac{TP+FN}{TP+FN+FP+TN}$

Figure 4.3: A simplified table.

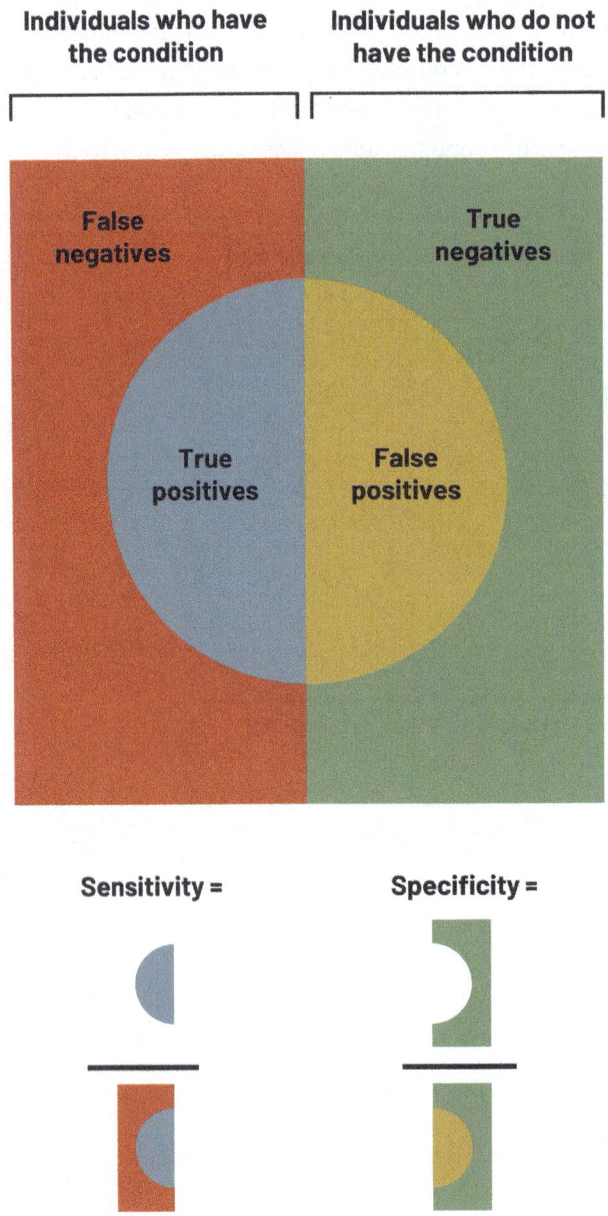

Figure 4.4: Sensitivity and specificity.

	Definition	Calculation
Sensitivity (true-positive rate)	The percent of positives identified by the screening tests that are truly positive. The higher this number, the more people we have correctly identified as having the outcome. It is calculated as the number of true positives (TP) over all tests that are positive according to the gold standard (TP+FN).	$\text{Sensitivity} = \frac{A}{A+C}$
Specificity (true-negative rate)	The percent of negatives identified by the screening test that are truly negative. The higher this number, the more people we have correctly identified as not having the outcome. It is calculated as the number of true negatives (TN) over all tests that are negative according to the gold standard (FP+TN).	$\text{Specificity} = \frac{D}{B+D}$
Positive predictive value (PPV)	The percent of positive results from the screening test that are true positives (TP). It is calculated as the number of TP over all tests that are positive according to the screening test (TP+FP).	$\text{Predictive value positive} = \frac{A}{A+B}$
Negative predictive value (NPV)	The percent of negative results from the screening test that are true negatives (TN). It is calculated as the number of TN over all tests that are negative according to the screening test (FN+TN).	$\text{Predictive value negative} = \frac{D}{C+D}$

Figure 4.5: Properties of validity tests.

Sensitivity and specificity are ***fixed*** properties of a test. They let us know how good a test is. No matter when the test is run, the sensitivity and the specificity will always be the same.

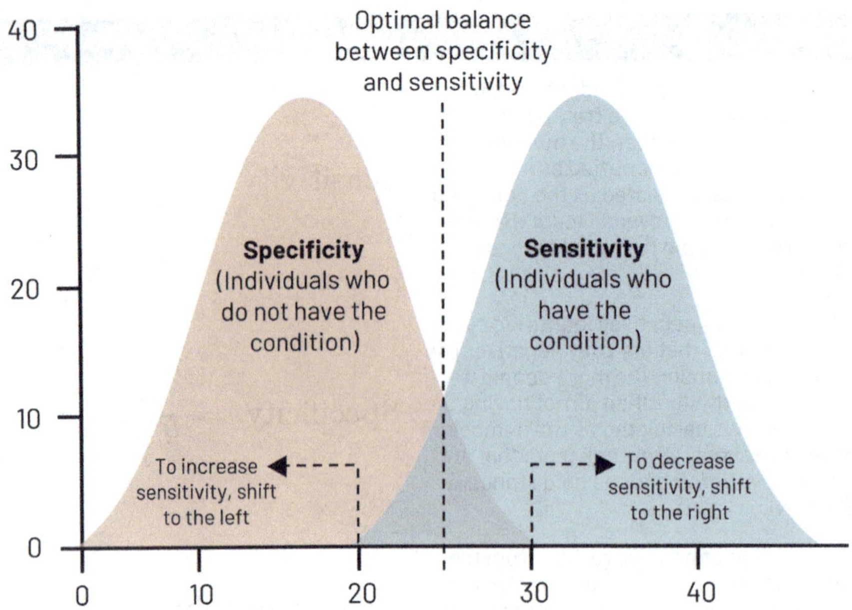

Figure 4.6: The optimization of sensitivity and specificity.

Looking at figure 4.6, there are two bell curves: one for patients without the disease (negatives) and those with the disease (positives). The black dotted line indicates the perfect balance of sensitivity and specificity—neither is 100 percent, but we have minimized both the number of false positives and the number of false negatives. If we move that dotted line to the left, we are increasing the number of positive cases that we identify (increase of sensitivity) at the expense of specificity. We have more false positives, but we are also doing a good job at ruling *out* disease. If we have a disease of high consequence like HIV or cancer, we want our test to have a really high sensitivity because we do not want to miss any possible cases. This does mean that some people will get false positives, so it is helpful to have a secondary test for verification. In the case of HIV, often people undergo rapid tests, and, if positive, then we will run confirmatory blood tests.

SnNOUT: When a highly **Sen**sitive test is **N**EGATIVE, it rules **OUT** disease.

If we move the dotted line to the right, we increase specificity at the expense of sensitivity. Specificity should be high for a screening test, but this can vary depending on whether you can afford a lot of misdiagnoses. If there is low stigma about a condition or the treatment is fairly benign, misdiagnoses are more acceptable to the population. For example, if you tell a patient who has a broken leg that it is *not* broken, harm can happen, and that is not acceptable. But if you tell a patient who does not have a broken finger that it needs to be splinted, the harm may be minimal: you can verify that it is not actually broken, and the splint can be removed. Highly specific tests are good at ruling *in* disease.

SpPIN: When a highly **Sp**ecific test is **P**OSITIVE, it rules **IN** disease.

Whereas sensitivity and specificity are fixed, PPV and NPV ***vary depending on disease prevalence*** in the population being tested. PPV and NPV let us know how to interpret our patient's test results.

- If prevalence of the disease is high, PPV is high and NPV is low.
- If prevalence of the disease is low (rare disease), PPV is low and NPV is high.

Beyond just sensitivity and specificity, it is important to know how much more likely a particular test result is going to be for people with the disease compared to those without the disease. This is called the **likelihood ratio** (figure 4.7). We can calculate the likelihood that a person with the disease tests positive compared to someone without the disease (**LR+**) and the likelihood that a person with the disease tests negative compared to someone without the disease (**LR-**). A LR+ that is greater than 10 indicates that the test is highly specific (very good at picking up negatives), whereas a LR- value of less than 0.1 indicates a highly sensitive test (very good at picking up positives). This is very important in clinical decision making.[6]

LR^+	Probability of **positive result** in patient with disorder / probability of **positive result** in patient without disorder	=	Sensitivity / 1-specificity	=	TP rate / FP rate	If $LR^+ > 10$, indicates a highly specific test
LR^-	Probability of **negative result** in patient with disorder / probability of **negative result** in patient without disorder	=	1-sensitivity / Specificity	=	FN rate / TN rate	If $LR^- < 0.1$, indicates a highly sensitive test

Figure 4.7: Likelihood ratio.

Further reading

SpPIN and SnNOUT are great mnemonic devices for remembering how to rule disease in or out, however there are caveats about using them in reality. This article by Pewsner et al. demonstrates how careful you should be when applying these principles.[7]

How do you improve sensitivity and specificity?

- Retrain the people doing the measurements. This reduces the amount of **misclassification** in tests that require human assessment.
- Recalibrate the screening instrument. This reduces the amount of imprecision in tools like scales.
- Use a different test.
- Use more than one test.
- Use visuals to help participants choose the answer that is valid for them.

Figure 4.8 shows examples of visuals that are more useful when trying to measure responses from patients because they remove some of the variability caused by subjective topics like pain.

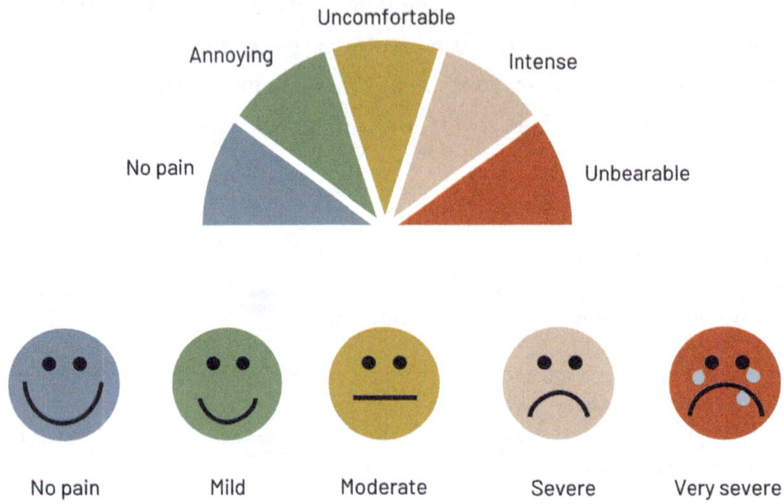

Figure 4.8: Examples of improved visuals.

Besides thinking in terms of calculations, it is important to know why false positives and false negatives are important in clinical medicine. In figure 4.9, we see two radiographs. In one, there is no deformity of the bone. If we told that patient they had a broken leg, we would be committing what is known as a **Type I error** (false positive). We need to either improve how we read the radiographs to stop making this type of mistake or we need to change who is reading them to avoid this mistake. In the second image, there is deformity of the bone. If we told that patient that they did not have a broken leg, we would be committing what is known as a **Type II error** (false negative). While the method we use to improve the chance we do not make a Type I error is the same as we might use in this case to not make a Type II error, the result of our error here would be more egregious: the patient clearly has a broken leg, and we would be delaying treatment. The patient may lose trust in the practitioner or, worse, suffer further damage.

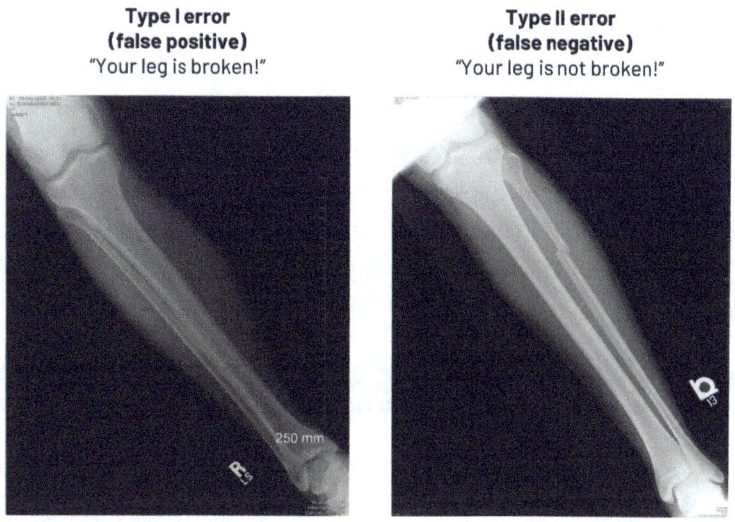

Figure 4.9: The importance of false positives and false negatives.

Example: PPV and NPV of the ImPACT Assessment[8]

If we want to see a real example of how the PPV and the NPV are used in clinical medicine, we can take a look at the ImPACT (Immediate Post-concussion Assessment and Cognitive Testing) tool. This tool is used to help identify whether athletes have post-concussive abnormalities after injury or not. Is this tool important in the arsenal against returning athletes to play too soon?

In a study of 122 athletes diagnosed with concussion and 70 athletes without recent concussion:

- 93 percent of athletes with a reliable increase in symptoms actually had concussion (PPV)
- 1 percent of athletes without a reliable increase in symptoms had a concussion (59 percent NPV)

How would you interpret these numbers?

Further reading

What kind of performance did RT-PCR have to detect SARS-CoV-2 in a hospital setting in 2020?[9]

How does the King-Devick test perform to identify concussion in collegiate athletes?[10]

4.5 Sources of Bias in Screening

There are several sources of bias in screening. **Lead time bias** is the perception that the screen-detected case has longer survival because the disease was identified early. **Length bias** is particularly relevant to cancer screening because tumors identified by screening are slower growing and have a better prognosis. **Selection bias** is when we make errors in how we select who is in our study. Because motivated participants (e.g., those with prior injury history) have a different probability of disease than do those who refuse to participate (e.g., those that have never been injured), we get biased study results.

Type	Definition	Examples	Strategies to reduce bias
Selection bias	Incorrectly picked the population to study. Results in a nonrepresentative study group.	Women and men with a family history are more likely to volunteer for a breast cancer study than people without a family history. These two groups have differing levels of risk.	• Randomize • Be strategic in where and how you recruit participants • Make sure your study population is representative of the group you want to make an inference about even if it means that you turn volunteers down • Example: Select patients with family history and some without and include family history as a part of the study to see the impact it makes on your answer
Lead-time bias	When earlier detection of the disease looks like it leads to increased survival over those that were not diagnosed earlier.	Two patients die at 68 years old of lung cancer. One was diagnosed at 50 with screening and the other started being symptomatic at 65.	• Adjust the survival time based on how severe disease is at the time of diagnosis. • Example: Patient A was Stage 1 at the time of diagnosis and Patient B was Stage 4 at the time of diagnosis. Find out whether each patient's length of survival was appropriate for the stage at diagnosis.
Length-time bias	Screening is more effective if the disease is latent longer compared to if the disease has a short latency period.	Patients with slow-growing tumors are in the majority of patients treated at your clinic, so you overestimate the length of survival for the rare patient with a fast-growing tumor.	• Randomize patients to determine the length of survival after screening compared to those that were not screened. • Example: Half of the patients in your clinic are randomized to being screened for tumors and half are not. You calculate the survival time for the two groups in your study to find differences to adjust your predictions.

Figure 4.10: Sources of bias in screening.

4.6 Natural History of Disease

A main reason to use a screening test is to identify disease earlier than we would without the test. However, a screening test is really useful only if there is something we can do to change the natural history of the disease. This means if we could increase survival, change the quality of life, eliminate disease better, or something similar.

In figure 4.11, we see a comparison between the expected trajectory of survival for a patient who is screened for disease compared to a patient who is not screened for disease. The disease begins at the same point for both patients (e.g., at 50 years of age). Both patients are asymptomatic at age 55, but one patient is screened at that time and is given a positive diagnosis. Treatment begins immediately. The other patient becomes symptomatic at age 60 and is diagnosed at that time. The first patient had 5 years of **lead time**, meaning more time to minimize the effect of the disease or slow its progression. Both patients die at 70 years of age. The patient who was not screened had 5 years of **survival time**, or time between diagnosis and death, whereas the patient who was screened had 10 years of **survival time**. In this particular example, screening did not lead to a longer survival, but it could have led to improved quality of life for the duration of the illness because we were able to potentially impact the natural history of the disease (e.g., slow the disease down, reverse the course of disease). Because both patients actually had disease at the same point and survived the same amount of time, their survival length after adjustment is the same. To assume otherwise would be to commit **lead time bias**. If instead the patient who was screened died at 75 instead of 70, that patient's survival actually would be different than the patient who was not screened. We would have a different impact on the natural history of disease: this patient had a longer survival and hopefully a better quality of life than the patient who was not screened. Both are indicators that screening is a good idea.

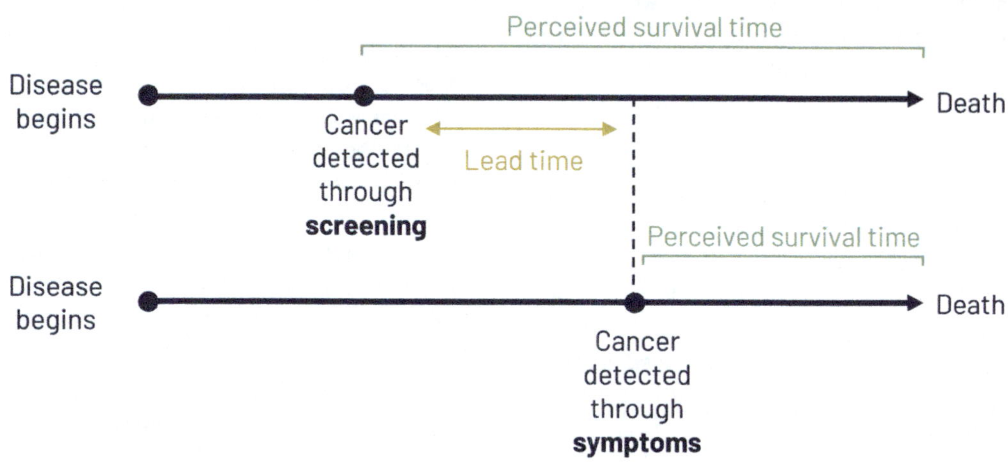

Figure 4.11: Natural history of disease.

Figure Descriptions

Figure 4.2: Above the table is condition according to gold standard (present or absent). Left of the table is test result (positive or negative). If present and positive, A. If absent and positive, B. If present and negative, C. If absent and negative, D. Reading left to right in the table: A, B, line break, C, D. Outside of the table are calculations for finding totals. Below the table left to right: total, A+C, B+D, line break, Sensitivity=A/(A+C). Specificity=D/(B+D). Right of the table top to bottom: total, A+B, C+D. Additional rightmost column: predictive value (+)=A/(A+B), predictive value (-)=C/(C+D). Grand total: A+B+C+D. Return to figure 4.2.

Figure 4.3: Above the table is disease (+) and disease (-). Left of the table is test (+) and test (-). If disease (+) and test (+), true positive. If disease (-) and test (+), false positive. If disease (+) and test (-), false negative. If disease (-) and test (-), true negative. Outside of the table are calculations for finding other values. Below the table left to right: sensitivity=TP/(TP+FN) and specificity=TN/(TN+FP). Right of the table top to bottom: predictive value (+)=TP/(TP+FP), predictive value (-)=TN/(TN+FN). Prevalence=(TP+FN)/(TP+FN+FP+TN). Return to figure 4.3.

Figure 4.4: True positives and false negatives make up every individual who have the condition. True negatives and false positives make up every individual who does not have the condition. Sensitivity=true positives/(true positives+false negatives). Specificity=true negatives/(true negatives+false positives). Return to figure 4.4.

Figure 4.6: Two overlapping bell curves representing specificity and sensitivity. X-axis and y-axis range from 0 to 40. Specificity bell curve (individuals who do not have the condition) is left of sensitivity (individuals who have the condition). The curves overlap slightly. Where they overlap is the optimal balance between specificity and sensitivity. To increase sensitivity, shift to the left. To decrease sensitivity, shift to the right. Return to figure 4.6.

Figure 4.7: Likelihood ratio (+)=probability of positive result in patient with disorder/probability of positive result in patient without disorder=sensitivity/(1-specificity)=TP rate/FP rate. If LR (+) > 10, indicates a highly specific test. Likelihood ratio (-)=probability of negative result in patient with disorder/probability of negative result in patient without disorder=(1-sensitivity)/specificity=FN rate/TN rate. If LR (-) < 0.1, indicates a highly sensitive test. Return to figure 4.7.

Figure 4.8: Rainbow of colors in a half circle with each color representing a point on the pain scale. Left to right: no pain (blue), annoying (green), uncomfortable (yellow), intense (pink), unbearable (red). A different pain scale is below, represented by 5 simple faces. Left to right: no pain (happy face), mild (slightly smiling face), moderate (neutral face), severe (sad face), very severe (crying). Return to figure 4.8.

Figure 4.9: Left: Example of Type I error (false positive). "Your leg is broken!" when the leg in the image is not broken. Right: Example of Type II error (false negative) "Your leg is not broken!" when the leg in the image is broken. Return to figure 4.9.

Figure 4.11: Two timelines. First: disease begins and cancer is detected through screening shortly after. Patient has a longer perceived survival time since cancer was detected early through screening (more lead time). Second: disease begins, more time passes, cancer is detected through symptoms. Patient has a shorter perceived survival time since cancer was detected later through symptoms. Lead time: The difference in time between the cancer being detected through screening versus symptoms. Return to figure 4.11.

Figure References

Figure 4.1: Precision and accuracy. Graphic by Kindred Grey. 2022. CC BY 4.0. Table data adapted under fair use from USMLE First Aid, Step 1.

Figure 4.2: The fourfold (2×2) table. Kindred Grey. 2022. CC BY 4.0.

Figure 4.3: A simplified table. Kindred Grey. 2022. CC BY 4.0.

Figure 4.4: Sensitivity and specificity. Kindred Grey. 2022. CC BY-SA 4.0. Adapted from *Sensitivity and Specificity 1.01* by FeanDoe, from WikimediaCommons (CC BY-SA 4.0).

Figure 4.5: Properties of validity tests. Adapted under fair use from USMLE First Aid, Step 1.

Figure 4.6: The optimization of sensitivity and specificity. Kindred Grey. 2022. CC BY 4.0.

Figure 4.7: Likelihood ratio. Kindred Grey. 2022. CC BY 4.0.

Figure 4.8: Examples of improved visuals. Kindred Grey. 2022. CC BY 4.0.

Figure 4.9: The importance of false positives and false negatives. Kindred Grey. 2022. CC BY-SA 2.0. Includes leg1 by Joe Goldberg, from Flickr (CC BY-SA 2.0) and Lower Leg Tib Fib Right x-ray 0000 no info, by Eric Schmuttenmaer, from WikimediaCommons (CC BY-SA 2.0).

Figure 4.10: Sources of bias in screening. Adapted under fair use from USMLE First Aid, Step 1.

Figure 4.11: Natural history of disease. Kindred Grey. 2022. CC BY 4.0. Adapted from Lead time bias by Mcstrother, from WikimediaCommons (CC BY 3.0).

Notes

1. Myerburg RJ, Vetter VL. Electrocardiograms should be included in preparticipation screening of athletes. Circulation. 2007;116(22):2616-2626.
2. Kligfield P, Gettes LS, Bailey JJ, et al. Recommendations for the standardization and interpretation of the electrocardiogram. Circulation. 2007;115(10):1306-1324.
3. Cleveland Clinic. Electrocardiogram (EKG). https://my.clevelandclinic.org/health/diagnostics/16953-electrocardiogram-ekg. Published 2022. Accessed 17 September 2023.
4. U.S. Preventive Services Task Force. Final Recommendation Statement. Cardiovascular disease risk: Screening With electrocardiography. https://www.uspreventiveservicestaskforce.org/uspstf/recommendation/cardiovascular-disease-risk-screening-with-electrocardiography. Published 2018. Accessed 17 September 2023.
5. Johns Hopkins Medicine. Electrocardiogram. https://www.hopkinsmedicine.org/health/treatment-tests-and-therapies/electrocardiogram. Published 2023. Accessed 17 September 2023.
6. Hayden SR, Brown MD. Likelihood ratio: A powerful tool for incorporating the results of a diagnostic test into clinical decisionmaking. *Ann Emerg Med*. 1999;33(5):575-580.
7. Pewsner D, Battaglia M, Minder C, Marx A, Bucher HC, Egger M. Ruling a diagnosis in or out with "SpPIn" and "SnNOut": A note of caution. *BMJ* (Clinical research ed). 2004;329(7459):209-213.
8. Van Kampen DA, Lovell MR, Pardini JE, Collins MW, Fu FH. The "value added" of neurocognitive testing after sports-related concussion. *Am J Sports Med*. 2006;34(10):1630-1635.
9. Brihn A, Chang J, K OY, et al. Diagnostic performance of an antigen test with RT-PCR for the detection of SARS-CoV-2 in a hospital setting—Los Angeles County, California, June-August 2020. *MMWR Morbidity and Mortality Weekly Report*. 2021;70(19):702-706.
10. Le RK, Ortega JD, Chrisman SPD, et al. King-Devick sensitivity and specificity to concussion in collegiate athletes. *J Athl Train*. 2023;58(2):97-105.

5. THE WRECKING BALL: BIAS, CONFOUNDING, INTERACTION AND EFFECT MODIFICATION

5.1 Sources of Study Errors

Studies will never be perfect. We start all of our work knowing this, but we should also control everything we can to make it the best it can be. We want a study with the best validity and reliability available. There are three things that can completely destroy or derail a study:

- **Bias**: A **systematic error** in how a study is designed.
- **Confounding**: A third related factor that distorts the relationship between exposure and outcome for all participants.
- **Interaction** and **effect modification**: Another third factor that distorts the relationship of exposure and outcome but does it differently for different participants.

Each of these concepts is better defined and explained on the following pages. Figure 5.1 shows us what could explain any association (e.g., a relative risk of 4.1 in a study) between a risk factor for disease and getting the disease. In statistics as in life, things can vary randomly. We might also see true causal associations. This is most often what we really want to see. For example, in the famous 1950 *British Medical Journal* paper "Smoking and Carcinoma of the Lung," Drs. Doll and Hill specifically showed a causal and temporal relationship between smoking and lung cancer.[1] This was one of the first times this was proven and has served as the basis for tobacco policy around the world. However, even in their article, Drs. Doll and Hill had to consider whether bias or confounding skewed their study results. They concluded that was not the case.

What can explain an association?	How can we look for or take care of it?
Random variability	Statistical precision estimates: p-value, confidence interval
Causal relationship	Bradford Hill criteria, randomization, regression, path analysis, rule out other possible explanations
Bias	Standardize questions, clear definitions, use objective data sources instead of or to supplement subjective data sources, plan ahead for attrition of participants, use validated measures
Confounding	Adjustment, restriction of study population, randomization, matching, regression
Interaction or effect modification	Present group specific results, restriction of study population

Figure 5.1: Possible explanations for an association between a risk factor and a disease.

You recall validity from chapter 4. When we are talking about designing and carrying out different studies, strong study validity comes down to how you planned each study.

- If you design it right and follow the right steps, your study is valid and will have unbiased results. On average, the results will be correct.
- If you do not design it right and/or do not follow the right steps, it will be invalid and have biased results. On average, the results will be incorrect.

5.1.1 Bias

Bias is a **systematic error** in how a study is designed. Bias results from a ***design error***, including the method of choosing participants or gathering information to define whether a participant has the exposure or disease. Bias is one thing that can alter the measure you created and make you think the answer to it is A when it is really B. This is also known as a false difference in a relationship between factors. As we can only do our own study, it is hard to determine whether our result is accurate. To determine if bias is confirmed to be present or how it may have influenced the answer we see would require infinite studies to see the truth. Instead we prevent bias best by:

- Using the appropriate study design
- Establishing valid and reliable methods of data collection
- Using appropriate analytic procedures

Most types of bias are either **selection** or **information** (figure 5.2):

- Selection: Error in how we picked participants
- Information: Error in how we obtain information (data) from participants

Types of bias can overlap, and rarely are we concerned with just one type of bias during a study. More specifically, **selection bias** is when individuals have different probabilities of being selected in the study sample according to their exposure and outcome. Selection bias means that the study does not have **external validity** (i.e., the results cannot be applied to any other population) and that the results will inaccurately represent the actual relationship being studied (i.e., compromised **internal validity**).

Information bias is when people systematically get placed in the wrong classification group for exposure and/or outcome (**misclassification**). When we make this mistake with everyone in the study, no matter their disease or exposure group, we consider it to be **non-differential**. Non-differential misclassification is when the misclassification of the exposure category is unrelated to the disease status and/or the misclassification of the disease category is unrelated to the exposure status.[2] When it makes a difference which group a subject is in (e.g., we only collect information incorrectly for controls), the bias is **differential**. Differential misclassification is when the misclassification of the exposure category is related to the disease status of the participant and/or if the misclassification of the disease status is related to the exposure category.[3] Information bias can also be failure to appropriately interpret the results or relationships seen in the data. Some people consider confounding to be a type of bias, so we have included it in figure 5.2. Misclassification can happen often in case-control and cohort studies. This concept is related to our prior discussion of **sensitivity, specificity, validity,** and **reliability**. If misclassification is present, we will not correctly calculate sensitivity or specificity. We also will have a false idea of the true validity or reliability of the answer from the study. Knowing how the misclassification or confounding occurs helps us decide what to do next analytically but certainly should involve a consultation with an epidemiologist or biostatistician to make sure the analysis is appropriate.

Type	Definition	Example
Selection Bias		
Selection bias	A bias that results in a sample population that is not representative of the population of interest and affects the internal validity of the study	Failure to confirm the age of participants prior to enrollment in the study results in needing to exclude 40 percent of the surveys captured
Volunteer bias / Self-selection bias	Those who volunteer for a study are clinically different than those who do not volunteer for the study.	People with a family history of cancer are more likely to volunteer for a study on breast cancer prevention.
Sampling bias	A bias that results in certain people having a greater chance of being selected than others and affects the external validity of the study	Choosing participants for a study of medical students by conveniently picking your friends to participate due to your relationship
Survivorship bias	A bias that results in only those who survived a disease being selected for a study	Patients who have few complications to COVID-19 may survive longer than patients who were hospitalized and so a study ten years later would capture people who had had milder disease.
Attrition bias	Participants who leave the study are different than the participants who stay.	Participants with comorbid conditions may leave the study early due to complications from those comorbidities, leaving the researcher with participants who have fewer comorbidities
Non-Response bias	Participants who do not respond to participate are different than the participants who choose to respond.	Participants who are older and less computer savvy are less likely to respond to requests by email to participate in a study.
Recall bias	Participants have difficulty remembering information or events from the past.	Patients may not recall whether they have ever had an exposure that is required to participate in the study.
Information Bias		
Performing study		
Recall bias	Participants have difficulty remembering information or events from the past.	Participants may not recall their blood type when asked and randomly select one that is incorrect.
Measurement bias	Data about the outcome, exposure, or other study factors are not accurately measured or categorized.	Study interviewers know a participant is an athlete and select "yes, concussion" no matter what the participant says.

Type	Definition	Example
Procedure bias	The administration of the study puts undue pressure on the participants, such as not enough time to complete a survey or too long a distance to complete a needed task. This could also mean that researchers or participants self-assign or nonrandomly assign people to study groups.	Participants at a factory are asked to fill out a survey about their supervisor in front of their supervisor at the beginning of a shift.
Observer-expectancy bias	Researchers influence respondents to answer a particular way to questions.	The researcher knows the patient is a case and asks the question in a way that suggests the correct answer is that there was an exposure.
Response bias	Participants are worried about social acceptability of their answer and may respond differently than is true.	Patients say that they eat 6–11 servings of fruits and vegetables daily when they actually eat fewer.
Interpreting results		
Confounding bias	A factor that makes you misinterpret the relationship between the exposure and the outcome	The association between teenage smoking and packaging/store placement is not independent of the influence of growing up seeing their parents smoke.
Lead-time bias	Disease is diagnosed earlier but the true course of disease is the same length as those who did not have early diagnosis.	Minoritized patients have breast cancer detected later than nonminoritized patients and appear to have a shorter life expectancy than those who have their cancer detected earlier.
Length-time bias	Disease that develops slowly is more likely to be detected early and have a better prognosis.	Slow-growing fibroids are able to be detected earlier at annual visits and monitored or removed compared to fast-growing fibroids.
Reading about the study		
Publication bias	When negative study results or very novel ideas are not published in favor of positive study results and "more interesting" topics	A manuscript is rejected by multiple journals for publication because none of the hypotheses was found to be true.

Figure 5.2: Bias.

In a textbook from the International Agency for Research on Cancer and the World Health Organization, dos Santos Silva provided a series of questions (figure 5.3) that researchers should ask themselves to determine whether selection or information bias exists in their study.[4] These questions should optimally be asked prior to study execution and regularly during the course of study implementation, analysis, and reporting. Chapter 13 of the *Cancer Epidemiology* text by dos Santos Silva[5] provides more detail on the importance of these questions and other factors to consider to minimize bias. Note that many questions about selection relate to making sure that the same procedures are used for enrolling participants in a study, the process does not differ based on who is doing the recruitment or the disease or exposure status of the participant, and that the **inclusion and exclusion criteria** are very clear. Both are necessary to best define who should be in the study population and who you actually want to exclude.

Inclusion criteria is a definitive list of characteristics of participants that you want to enroll in the study and can be very minimal or very detailed. For example:

1. Children who go to Alpha Elementary School
2. Children between the ages of five and seven who go to Alpha Elementary School, are in kindergarten or first grade, have lived in town Alpha since birth, and who bring their own lunch to school

Exclusion criteria is a list of characteristics that participants should not have. These can also be minimal or very detailed. For example:

1. Children in town Alpha who attend any school other than Alpha Elementary School at the present time
2. Children younger than five or older than seven years, children who were not born in town Alpha or have not lived in town Alpha their entire lives, and children who eat prepared school meals or do not eat meals

Selection bias	• Was the study population clearly defined? • What were the inclusion and exclusion criteria? • Were refusals, losses to follow-up, etc., kept to a minimum? • In cohort and intervention studies: Were the groups similar except for the exposure/intervention status? Was the follow-up adequate? Was it similar for all groups? • In case-control studies: Did the controls represent the population from which the cases arose? Was the identification and selection of cases and controls influenced by their exposure status?
Measurement bias	• Were the measurements as objective as possible? • Were the measurements as objective as possible? • Were the subjects and observers blind? • Were the observers and interviewers rigorously trained? • Were clearly written protocols used to standardize procedures in data collection? • Were the study subjects randomized to observers or interviewers? • Was information provided by the patient validated against any existing records? • Were the methods used for measuring the exposure(s) and outcome(s) of interest (e.g., questionnaire, laboratory assays) validated?
Were strategies built into the study design to allow assessment of the likely direction and magnitude of the bias?	

Figure 5.3: How to check for bias in epidemiological studies.

One way to minimize selection bias is called **case-based control selection**. People who participate in health screenings such as mammograms are generally different from people who do not participate in these health screenings. They are more likely to have characteristics that are different (e.g., family history of disease or age), so comparing them to other people is akin to comparing apples and oranges. If we select our controls from the same pool of people that cases come from (i.e., case-based controls), the two groups will be more similar (e.g., Granny Smith apples compared to Gala apples). Our next example shows how we might avoid selection and information bias using case-based control selection.

Example: Selection bias and information bias avoidance

We want to do a study about long-term effects of ankle injuries from sport. As we work to define our specific study population, we think we want to select participants from emergency (ER) records. If we are not more specific about our study, we will have bias in our participant selection because our study answer will not apply to all people with ankle injuries from sport, just those who are seen in the ER. From what we know about SRI, people who go to the ER are more likely to have more severe injuries than those who do not go to the ER. They are also much more likely to have health insurance than those who do not go to the ER.

If the severity of the ankle injury is the same in the population that seeks treatment at the ER as in the population that did not seek treatment at the ER, there is limited selection bias due to where our cases come from. Severity is not the deciding factor in where to seek treatment.

However, because people are likely to select where and how they get treatment due to the severity of the injury, there is going to be selection bias in our study. To reduce the problem, we should reframe our research question to be *the long-term effects of ankle injuries from sport that seek treatment in the ER*. We selected a specific population. We might still end up with bias in our study, but the effect of it is lessened. This is also known as **compensating bias**, or the attempt to equalize the bias in the populations being compared (e.g., choosing to compare patients in the ER to other patients in the ER rather than those outside of the ER).

We further define our inclusion and exclusion criteria, then prepare the questions for participants. We choose to use a survey to ask participants in the ER about the grade of ankle sprain they had the first time they sprained their ankle. If asked the question exactly that way, participants who are in the ER with their first ankle sprain will be able to better recall the grade because that information is new and fresh. However, patients who have had multiple ankle sprains or a long time span between sprains may struggle to recall and will likely be misclassified. We can avoid this type of information bias by providing either different and larger categories for patients to pick from (e.g., "I could not walk on it" or "I needed surgery") or even potentially selecting patients from the hospital for whom you can obtain prior records to verify their grade sprain. Either of these solutions can introduce biases of their own, making it an important decision to plan out.

5.1.2 Confounding

Confounding is a third factor that makes you misinterpret the relationship you see between an exposure and an outcome. The confounder is unequally distributed across the population. The type of influence it has affects everyone involved the same way.

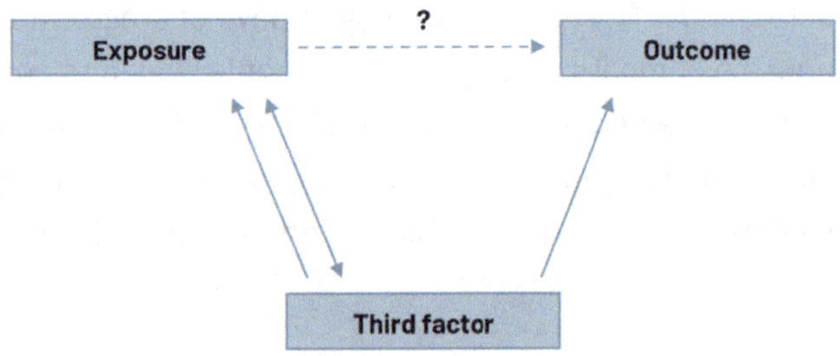

Figure 5.4: Definition of confounding.

Unlike bias, confounding is a real factor in the relationship between the exposure and the outcome. In order to be a confounder, a factor has to meet three criteria:

1. It has to not be in the causal pathway. This means the exposure does not lead to this factor and then leads to the outcome.
2. It has to be related to both the exposure and the outcome. The relationship to the exposure could be causal (the third factor causes the exposure) or it could be noncausal (the third factor and the exposure are related, but one doesn't cause the other). The relationship to the outcome has to be causal (the confounder has to cause the outcome).
3. The distribution of the factor among comparison groups has to be unequal. If the level of this factor was the same for everyone, there is no confounding because the influence in the two groups cannot be different (1 = 1).

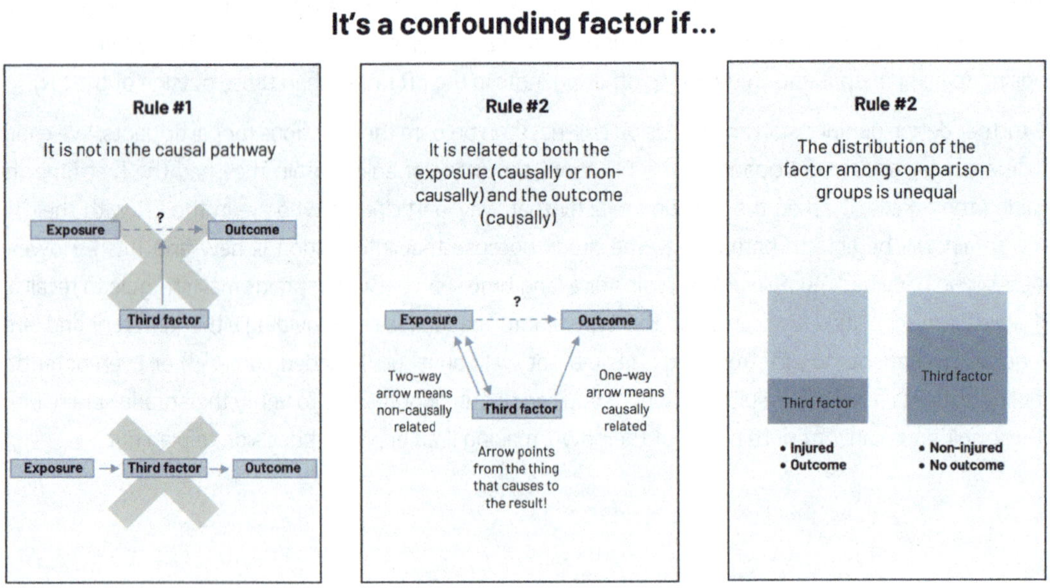

Figure 5.5: What is a confounder?

Any risk factor can be a confounder but it can't be caused by the disease, it doesn't have to be a causal risk factor, and it has to predict the future development of the disease. How do you find confounders?

- Find a subject matter expert.
- Look at the literature.
- Think outside the box.
- Draw out all the possible causal relationships using a **Directed Acyclic Graph** (DAG) or the **web of causation** or a similar tool. Both are conceptual representations of a series of relationships.

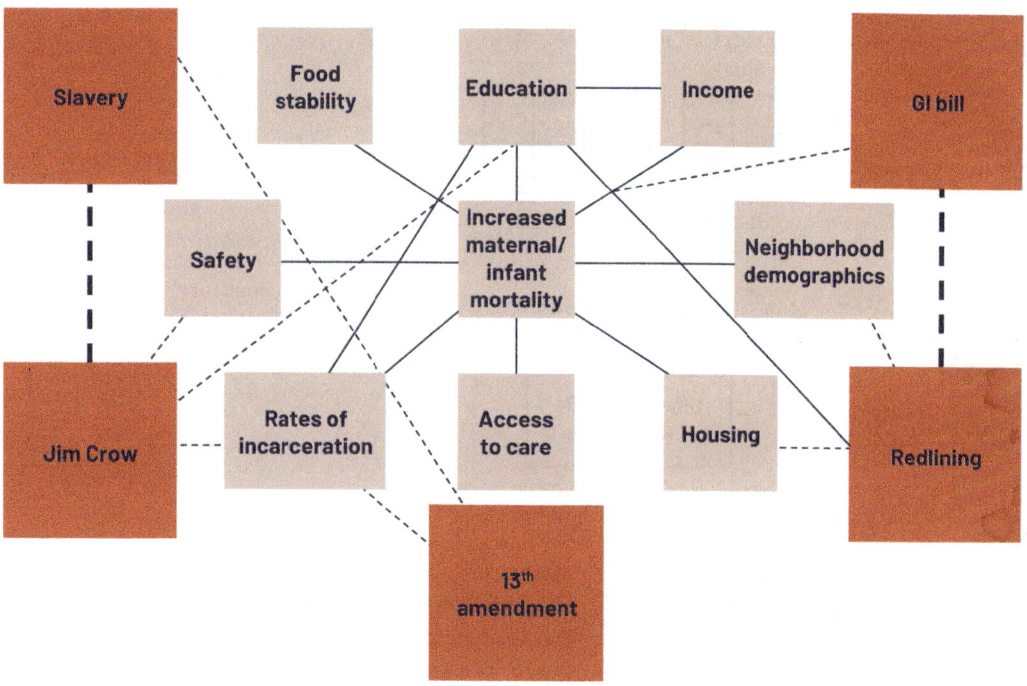

Figure 5.6: Web of causation example of the SDOH. (Web of causation: example of the structural and social determinants' impact on health).

5.1.2.1 Assessing for Confounding

You can **assess** (i.e., look for) the presence of confounding using a tool called **stratification** (figure 5.7). Stratification allows us to look at how our answer changes depending on the comparison groups. You can also use stratification to **control for** or **adjust** for (i.e., take care of) confounding. Other methods are restriction, matching, and regression. Some of the methods can be used prior to the study (design) and some can be used while you are completing your analysis.

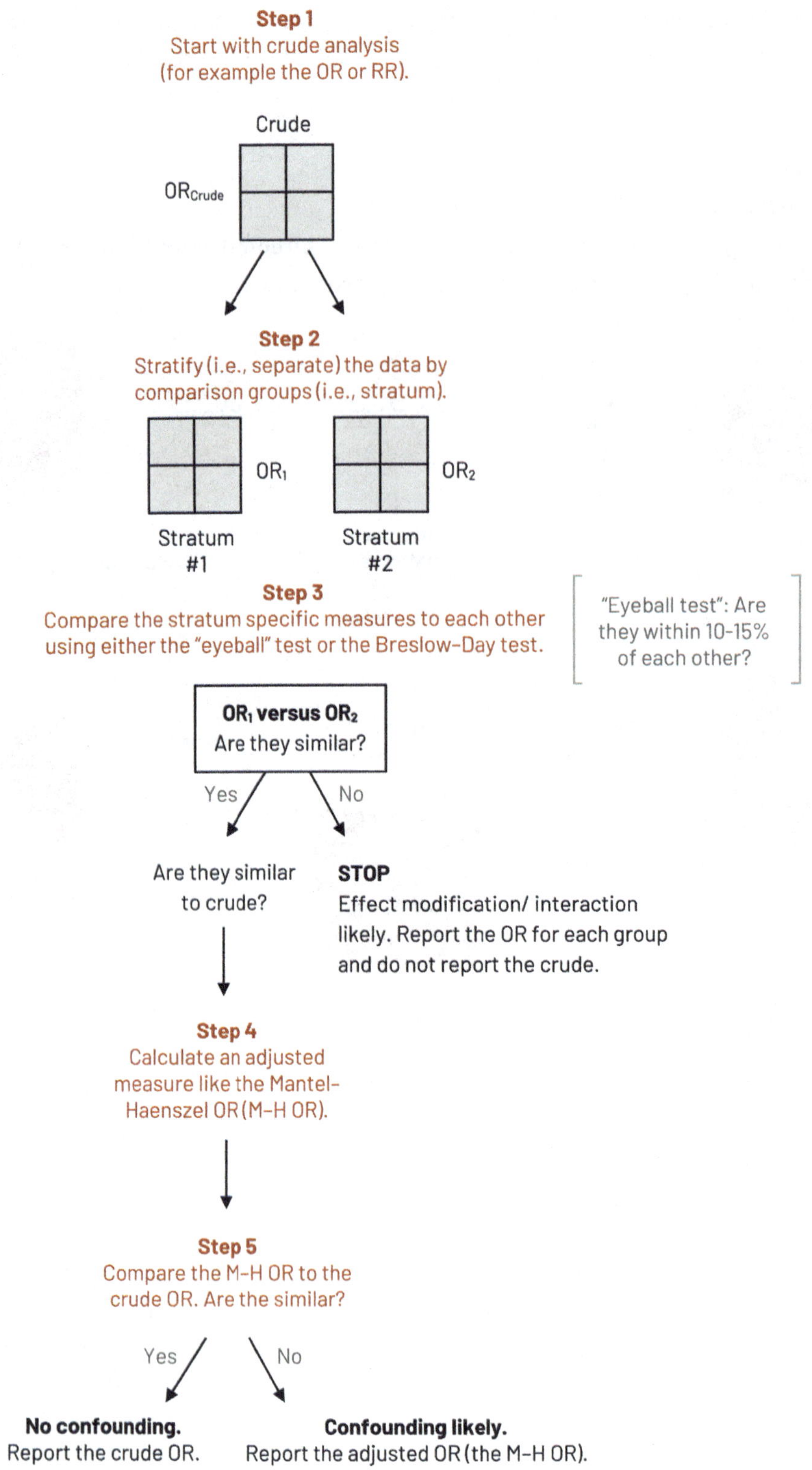

Figure 5.7: Stratification steps.

Let's walk through an example of how we might use stratification to see how family income influences the relationship between school sport participation and ankle sprains.

Example: Stratification

Step one of stratification is to calculate the measure of association, just as shown in chapter 3. The measure considers only the relationship between the exposure and the outcome, so it is considered to be **crude** or **unadjusted**. Let's say we find that there is a positive relationship between school sport participation and ankle sprains (ORcrude = 3.2). Because we need to consider the effect of a third variable on this relationship, we must take that third factor into account at this point. Before we get here, we should have already made sure that this third factor even qualifies as a potential confounding variable. Our comparison groups in this example are people with family income above $100,000 a year (high) and people with a family income at or below $100,000 a year (low).

In **Step two**, we need to calculate the same measure of association we just calculated in step one but separately for people with a high family income (stratum # 1) and then with a low family income (stratum # 2). We find out that people with a high family income have a high odds for ankle sprain with school sport participation (ORhigh income = 4.0) but so do those with a low income (ORlow income = 3.8).

In **Step three** we need to compare these estimates to each other and then the crude. If we use the **"eyeball method,"** meaning we look to see if the numbers are about 10 percent different from each other, we can easily find out that 10 percent of 4.0 is 0.4. Is the value of 3.8 in the range of 4.0 – 0.4 and 4.0 + 0.4?

$$4.0 - 0.4 = 3.6$$

$$4.0 + 0.4 = 4.4$$

The value 3.8 is in the range of 3.6 to 4.4. We say that the stratum-specific odds ratios are similar because of this. There is a statistical test we could have used called the **Breslow-Day Test**, but it is beyond the scope of this text. That test can be easily calculated by most software.

We not only want to see if the stratum-specific numbers are similar to each other, we also want to see if they are similar to the crude OR. The crude OR is outside of the range we just calculated, so we know it is different than the estimate for people with high incomes.

$$3.8 - 0.38 = 3.42$$

$$3.8 + 0.38 = 4.18$$

The crude OR is also outside of the range for the estimate for people with low income. This means we can proceed to our next step. If we had found that the crude OR was similar to both stratum-specific estimates, we would stop here and say confounding is unlikely. There does not seem to be any influence of the third variable on the relationship between school sport participation and ankle sprains. However, if it was similar to one but not the other, we would still continue with our steps to assess for confounding, though perhaps with a little less confidence that it is present. Finally, if the stratum-specific measures were not similar to each other, especially if they were on opposite sides of the crude estimate, we would stop here and say that confounding is not likely, but effect modification or interaction is likely. We would ignore the crude estimate and move forward to discussing just the stratum-specific estimates.

In **Step four** we calculate a measure that pools together the stratum but in a way to still take into account that the groups are for high income and low income. Many times we calculate the Mantel-Haenszel (M-H) estimate (this can be for OR, RR, or other measures). In this example, we would calculate the M-H OR. This is a new version of the OR that includes all three factors. Say we find that the M-H OR in this example is 3.9.

In **Step five** we then compare our M-H OR to the crude OR. If they are similar, confounding is likely not present and the third factor does not influence the relationship between our exposure and outcome. If they are different, confounding likely is present, and we use only this adjusted measure from now on.

$$3.9 - 0.39 = 3.51$$

$$3.9 + 0.39 = 4.29$$

Is the crude OR of 3.2 in the range of 3.51 to 4.29? No. Because of this, we say that confounding is present. Family income confounds the relationship between school sport participation and ankle sprains. We might report this by saying there is a positive association between school sport participation and ankle sprains when adjusting for family income (M-H OR = 3.9).

5.1.3 Interaction and Effect Modification

Interaction and **effect modification** are similar and the terms are often used interchangeably, but they are actually very different concepts. Why do we tend to use the terms interchangeably? How are these things similar? They both refer to a third factor that influences the relationship of the exposure and outcome but is different for different people. However, there is a big difference about why the relationship is different.

- **Effect modification** is when the effect of the exposure on the outcome is modified by the level of a third factor (the effect modifier/control variable)
    - Biological interaction
        - Antagonism and synergy
    - Definition is based on homogeneity and heterogeneity
- **Interaction** is when the observed joint effect of a risk factor and the third factor is greater than expected effect from the individual effects
    - Statistical interaction
        - Additive and multiplicative

In very simple terms, the difference between effect modification and interaction is biology versus statistics. As you read journal articles, know that the terms are used interchangeably, so be careful about how you interpret the results. We use interaction and effect modification to identify differences and disparities in health outcomes between groups of people. We can find out what groups of people have a much higher risk of developing disease or having a poor outcome compared to others. Effect modification is also an important consideration in pharmacology when you consider how two drugs or treatments might interact with each other.

Example: Effect modification

Men and women can develop breast cancer. If we found out that the odds of developing breast cancer if someone lives in the United States is 8.3 (OR_{crude} = 8.3), we might think that everyone needed the same level of intervention. However, biology plays a role in how breast cancer develops and who it develops in. If we stratify our population by sex, we might see that people assigned female at birth have an OR of 12.3 and that those assigned male at birth have an OR of 2.5. These are very different risk profiles based on sex at birth, and they completely change how we might proceed with interventions or even simple discussions with our patients. It may affect our choice of treatment and prevention methods. If we follow our rules of stratification (section 5.1.2), we stop here and say that confounding does not appear to be present by sex but that we see effect modification. We might say that the probability of developing breast cancer is higher for people assigned female at birth that live in the United States than those that live elsewhere (OR_{women} = 12.3). People assigned female at birth have a higher probability of breast cancer than people assigned male at birth, but people assigned male at birth living in the United States also have a higher probability of developing breast cancer compared to those that live elsewhere (OR_{men} = 2.5).

5.2 Summary

Keep **bias** to a minimum by setting guidelines for your study and sticking to them.

- Be careful about who you select.
- Be careful about who you compare your subjects to.
- Be careful how you collect information so you don't misclassify.

Confounding is real. Think about all possible relationships in your data as you design and analyze your information. Failing to do so will result in erroneous conclusions. **Interaction** and **effect modification** can help us see if there are patients who will benefit from a particular therapy. If you know this exists, do not combine the groups that are different or you will have errors in analysis and interpretation.

Figure Descriptions

Figure 5.4: Three boxes form upside down triangle shape. Top left box: exposure. Top right box: outcome. Bottom center box: third factor. Third factor points to exposure and outcome. Exposure points back to third factor. Question mark above arrow that points from exposure to outcome. Return to figure 5.4.

Figure 5.5: It's a confounding factor if…Rule #1: It is not in the causal pathway. Model crossed out with an X indicating that third factor does not influence the exposure or outcome. Rule #2: It is related to both the exposure (causally or non-causally) and the outcome (causally). Two way arrow means non-causally related. Arrow points from the thing that causes to the result! One-way arrow means causally related. Rule #3: The distribution of the factor among comparison groups is unequal. Left: bar graph that shows the third factor as skewed to be around one-third, either injured or outcome. Right: chart that shows the third factor as skewed to be around two thirds of the bar, either non-injured or no outcome. Return to figure 5.5.

Figure 5.6: Theoretical framework used to identify structural and social determinants of maternal and infant mortality in the United States. Structural determinants (slavery, GI bill, Jim Crow, 13th amendment, redlining) shape the distribution of social determinants (food stability, education, income, safety, rates of incarceration, access to care housing, neighborhood demographics). The multiple and interconnected pathways between structural and social determinants lead to increased maternal and infant mortality rates and socially defined inequities in these outcomes. Return to figure 5.6.

Figure 5.7: Step 1: Start with crude analysis (for example the OR or RR represented in 2×2 table with labels crude and OR sub crude). Step 2: Stratify (i.e., separate) the data by comparison groups (i.e., stratum). Two 2×2 tables. Left table is OR1 and stratum 1. Right table is OR2 and stratum 2. Step 3: Compare the stratum specific measures to each other using either the eyeball test (are they within 10-15% of each other?) or the Breslow-Day test. If OR1 and OR2 are not similar, stop (Effect modification/interaction likely. Report the OP for each group and do not report the crude.) If OR1 and OR2 are similar, and they are similar to crude, proceed to step 4. Step 4: Calculate an adjusted measure like the Mantel-Haenszel OR (M-H OR). Step 5: Compare the M-H OR to the crude OR. If they are similar, no confounding (Report the crude OR). If they are not similar, confounding is likely (Report the adjusted OR, the M-H OR). Return to figure 5.7.

Figure References

Figure 5.1: Possible explanations for an association between a risk factor and a disease. Adapted under fair use from USMLE First Aid, Step 1. Gianicolo EAL, Eichler M, Muensterer O, Strauch K, Blettner M. Methods for evaluating causality in observational studies. *Dtsch Arztebl Int*. 2020;116(7):101-107. Pannucci CJ, Wilkins EG. Identifying and avoiding bias in research. *Plast Reconstr Surg*. 2010;126(2):619-625. Kestenbaum B. Methods to control for confounding. In: *Epidemiology and Biostatistics: An Introduction to Clinical Research*. Springer New York; 2009:101-111. Corraini P, Olsen M, Pedersen L, Dekkers OM, Vandenbroucke JP. Effect modification, interaction and mediation: An overview of theoretical insights for clinical investigators. *Clin Epidemiol*. 2017;9:331-338.

Figure 5.2: Bias. Adapted under fair use from USMLE First Aid, Step 1.

Figure 5.3: How to check for bias in epidemiological studies. Adapted and used for noncommercial education according to IARC terms of use from IARC and dos Santos Silva I. Interpretation of epidemiological studies. In. Cancer epidemiology: principles and methods: IARC; 1999:277-303.

Figure 5.4: Definition of confounding. Kindred Grey. 2022. CC BY 4.0.

Figure 5.5: What is a confounder? Kindred Grey. 2022. CC BY 4.0.

Figure 5.6: Web of causation example of the SDOH. Adapted with permission from J. Roach, 2016. *Web of Causation*. CC BY NC-SA 4.0.

Figure 5.7: Stratification steps. Kindred Grey. 2022. CC BY 4.0.

Notes

1. Doll R, Hill AB. Smoking and carcinoma of the lung. *BMJ* (Clinical research ed). 1950;2(4682):739-748.
2. Department of Epidemiology at the Columbia University Mailman School of Public Health, Center for New Media Teaching and Learning. Epiville: Bias Data Analysis Questions. https://epiville.ccnmtl.columbia.edu/bias/data_analysis_questions.html. Published 2022. Accessed 2022.
3. Department of Epidemiology at the Columbia University Mailman School of Public Health, Center for New Media Teaching and Learning. Epiville: Bias Data Analysis Questions. https://epiville.ccnmtl.columbia.edu/bias/data_analysis_questions.html. Published 2022. Accessed 2022.
4. dos Santos Silva I. Interpretation of epidemiological studies. In. Cancer epidemiology: principles and methods: IARC; 1999:277-303.
5. dos Santos Silva I. Interpretation of epidemiological studies. In. Cancer epidemiology: principles and methods: IARC; 1999:277-303.

STUDY GUIDE: MEASURING THINGS IN EPIDEMIOLOGY

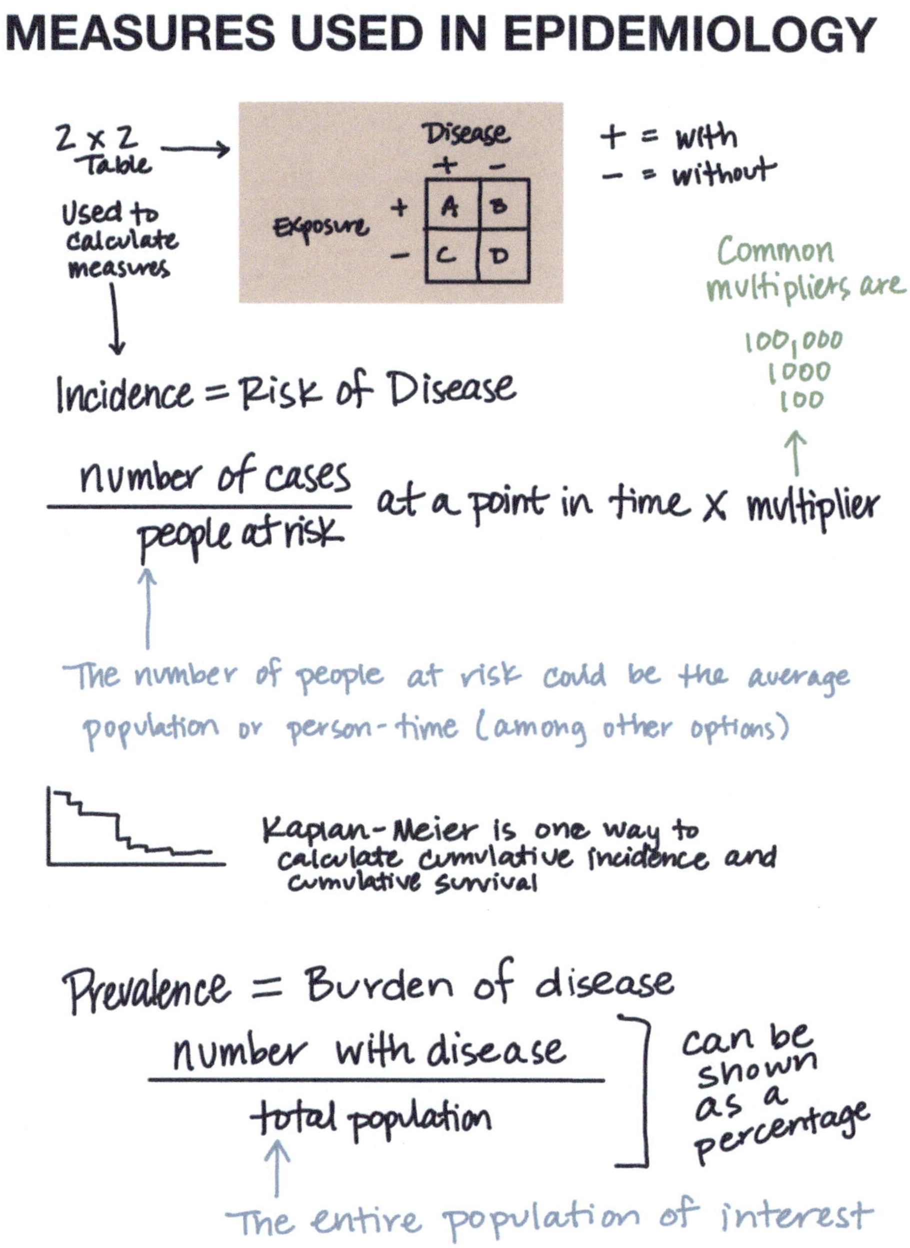

STUDY GUIDE: STUDY DESIGNS

MEASURES USED IN EPIDEMIOLOGY

2 x 2 Table →

Used to calculate measures

		Disease +	Disease −
Exposure	+	A	B
	−	C	D

+ = with
− = without

#1 Incidence = Risk of Disease

$$\frac{\text{number of cases}}{\text{people at risk}} \text{ at a point in time} \times \text{multiplier}$$

Common multipliers are
100,000
1000
100

The number of people at risk could be the average population or person-time (among other options)

Incidence can be used to calculate:

1A Relative risk (Risk Ratio)

$$RR = \frac{A/A+B}{C/C+D}$$

	D+	D−	Total
E+	A	B	A+B
E−	C	D	C+D

1B Relative risk reduction

$$RRR = 1 - RR$$

1C Risk Difference (RD) = Attributable Risk (AR)

RD = AR = A/A+B − C/C+D

1D Attributable Risk %

$$AR\% = \frac{A/A+B - C/C+D}{A/A+B} \times 100$$

1E Absolute Risk Reduction

ARR = C/C+D − A/A+B or $\frac{RR-1}{RR}$

1F Number needed to treat

NNT = 1/ARR

1G Number needed to harm

NNH = 1/AR

#2 An alternative to the incidence rate is the Attack rate

$$\text{Attack rate} = \frac{\text{Number that ate the food and got sick}}{\text{Total that ate the food}} \times 100$$

#3 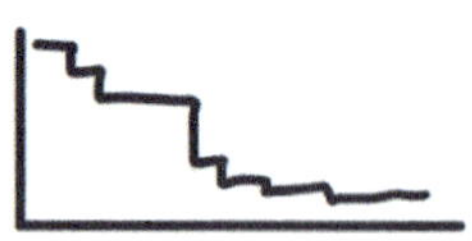 Kaplan-Meier is one way to calculate cumulative incidence and cumulative survival

#4 Prevalence = Burden of disease

$$\frac{\text{number with disease}}{\text{total population}}$$

can be shown as a percentage

↑ total population: The entire population of interest

Prevalence can be used to calculate:

3A Prevalence rate ratio

$$PRR = \frac{A / A+B}{C / C+D}$$

3B Population attributable risk

$$PAR = \frac{AR}{\dfrac{\text{Total exposed}}{\text{Total population}}}$$

or more simply:

$|AR\%| \times \text{Prevalence}$

	D+	D-	Total
E+	A	B	A+B
E-	C	D	C+D
Total	A+C	B+D	A+B+C+D

3C Population Attributable Risk %

$$\frac{AR}{(A+B) \times \left[\dfrac{A+C}{N}\right]} \times 100$$

Measures of Association

Incidence can be used to calculate:

Relative risk (Risk Ratio)

$$RR = \frac{A / A+B}{C / C+D}$$

	D+	D-	Total
E+	A	B	A+B
E-	C	D	C+D

$$\frac{A}{A+B}$$ = Incidence of disease in the exposed

$$\frac{C}{C+D}$$ = Incidence of disease in the unexposed

This means the relative risk is the risk of disease in the exposed relative to the risk of disease in the unexposed.

We use the relative risk as our first choice in a cohort study.

COHORT

The O and O are alike so they are relatives!

If you imagine the Os in COHORT as eyes...

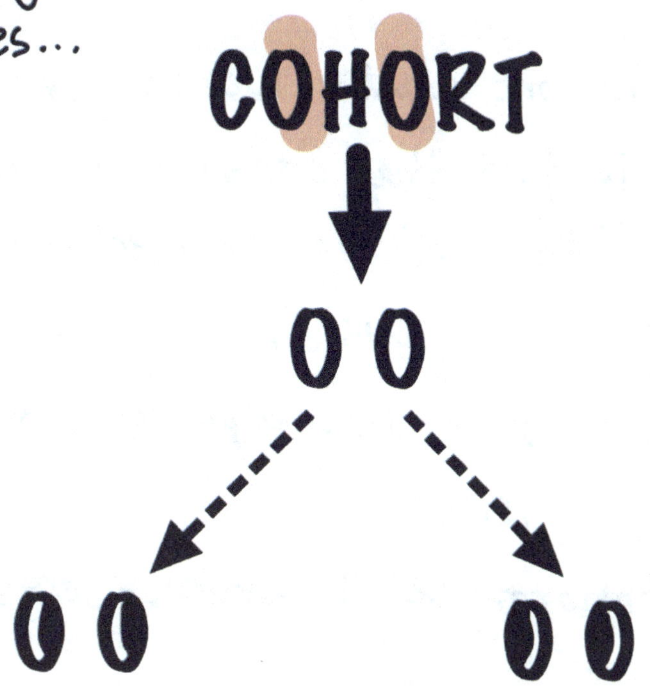

Prospective Cohort

Look forward to see what happens

Retrospective cohort

Look back to see what happens

Our goal is to start with knowledge of exposure and find the occurence of disease

The odds ratio is also a choice to calculate in a cohort study. The reason and method is different than how we use it in a case control study.

In a cohort study, we use the odds ratio to find the odds (or chance or probability) of an exposed person developing the disease compared to the odds of a non-exposed person developing disease.

In a cohort, RCT, cross-sectional, etc:

	D+	D-	Total
E+	A	B	A+B
E-	C	D	C+D

$\frac{A}{A+B}$ = chance of disease in the exposed

$\frac{B}{A+B}$ = chance of no disease in the exposed

$$\frac{A/A+B}{B/A+B} = \frac{A}{\cancel{A+B}} \cdot \frac{\cancel{A+B}}{B} = \frac{A}{B}$$ = odds of disease in the exposed

	D+	D-	Total
E+	A	B	A+B
E-	C	D	C+D

$$\frac{C}{C+D} = \text{chance of disease in the unexposed}$$

$$\frac{D}{C+D} = \text{chance of no disease in the unexposed}$$

$$\frac{C/C+D}{D/C+D} = \frac{C}{\cancel{C+D}} \cdot \frac{\cancel{C+D}}{D} = \frac{C}{D} = \text{odds of disease in the unexposed}$$

$$\frac{A/B}{C/D} = \frac{\text{odds of disease in the exposed}}{\text{odds of disease in the unexposed}}$$

$$OR = \frac{A/B}{C/D} = \frac{A}{B} \cdot \frac{D}{C} = \frac{AD}{BC} = \text{cross product ratio}$$

As you can see, this equation is a ratio of odds. In particular, this is called the **odds ratio of disease** and is used instead of the relative risk when the outcome (disease) is ~10% of the population or less (rare).

If we are using a case-control study, we calculate the OR differently.

Case-control

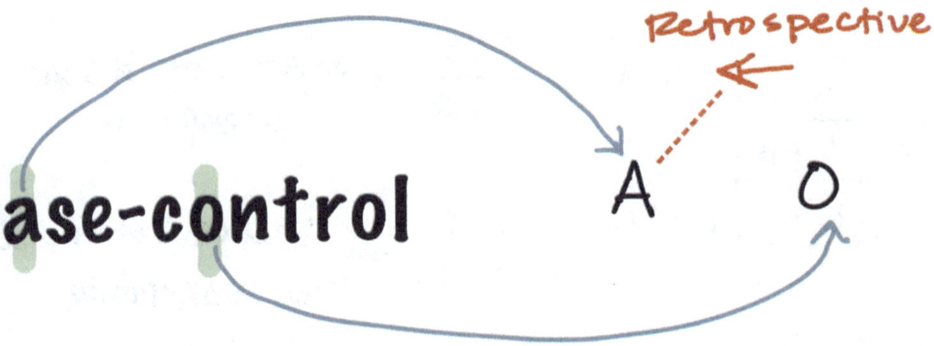

The first vowels are at <u>odds</u> with each other → odds ratio

A comes before O

Cases come before controls

Pick cases (diseased) people then pick controls (non-diseased) people

Our goal is to start with knowledge of disease and find the most likely exposure that caused disease

When we calculate the odds ratio in a case-control study, we are calculating the odds ratio of exposure. What is the chance that a particular exposure is associated with the disease?

	D+	D-
E+	A	B
E-	C	D
Total	A+C	B+D

$$\frac{A}{A+C} = \text{chance of exposure in the diseased}$$

$$\frac{C}{A+C} = \text{chance of no exposure in the diseased}$$

$$\frac{A/A+C}{C/A+C} = \frac{A}{\cancel{A+C}} \cdot \frac{\cancel{A+C}}{C} = \frac{A}{C} = \text{odds of exposure in the diseased}$$

	D+	D-
E+	A	B
E-	C	D
Total	A+C	B+D

$$\frac{B}{B+D} = \text{chance of exposure in the nondiseased}$$

$$\frac{D}{B+D} = \text{chance of no exposure in the nondiseased}$$

$$\frac{B/B+D}{D/B+D} = \frac{B}{\cancel{B+D}} \cdot \frac{\cancel{B+D}}{D} = \frac{B}{D} = \text{odds of exposure in the nondiseased}$$

$$\frac{A/C}{B/D} = \frac{\text{odds of exposure in the diseased}}{\text{odds of exposure in the nondiseased}}$$

$$OR = \frac{A/C}{B/D} = \frac{A}{C} \cdot \frac{D}{B} = \frac{AD}{BC} = \text{cross product ratio}$$

The OR is the only measure we can calculate with the case-control because of how we identify the study population

STUDY GUIDE: DIAGNOSTICS AND SCREENING

Screening Tests

New Test	Gold Standard +	Gold Standard −
+	A	B
−	C	D

=

New Test	Gold Standard +	Gold Standard −
+	TP	FP
−	FN	TN

True Positive — TP = actually positive + your test agrees
False Positive — FP = actually negative + your test disagrees
False Negative — FN = actually positive + your test disagrees
True Negative — TN = actually negative + your test agrees

A) How good is the test? Sensitivity and Specificity

1) sensitivity – Is the test good at detecting disease?

very important if you need to rule disease out!

SENSITIVITY → SNOUT

If sensitivity is high, you are confident that your test accurately captures all the positives so a negative isn't likely to be really positive. Rule it OUT!

Gold Standard

New Test	+	−
+	TP (A)	FP (B)
−	FN (C)	TN (D)

$$\text{Sensitivity} = \frac{TP}{TP+FN}$$

Also seen as

$$\frac{A}{A+C}$$

2) specificity – Is the test good at detecting when there is no disease?

Very important when you need to rule disease IN!

SPECIFICITY → SPIN

If specificity is high, you are confident that your test accurately captures all the negatives so a positive isn't likely to be really negative. Rule it IN!

		Gold Standard +	Gold Standard −
New Test	+	TP (A)	FP (B)
	−	FN (C)	TN (D)

$$\text{Specificity} = \frac{TN}{TN+FP}$$

Also seen as

$$\frac{D}{B+D}$$

3) The relationship between sensitivity and specificity

BALANCE BETWEEN THE TWO

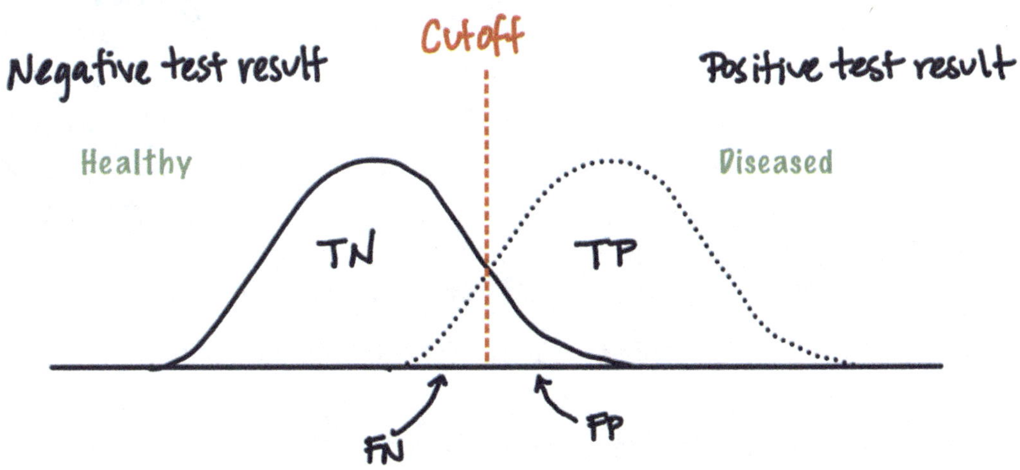

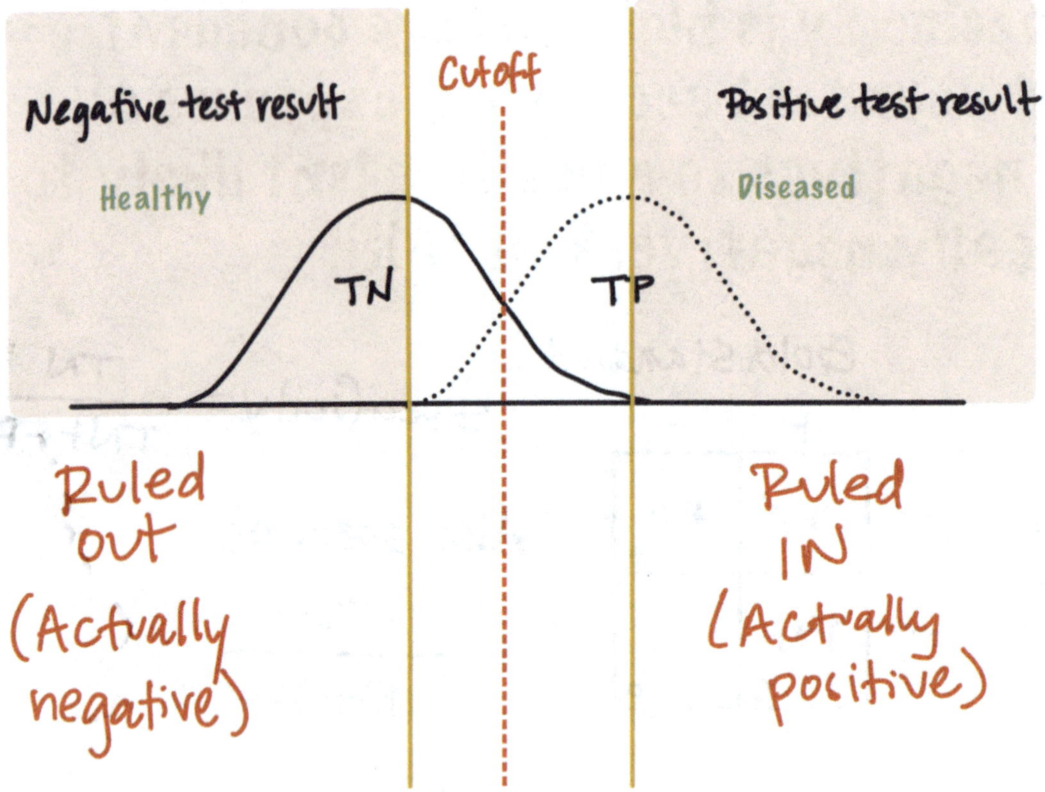

Happy Medium

More important to identify those with a concussion but not at the expense of having people overdiagnosed.

You have false positives AND false negatives.

If incorrect dx harms people, balance is key (ex: test in utero for birth defect)

If + there is a chance you are −.

If − there is a chance you are +.

Test is mostly valid and reliable.

Optimally, you want 100% sensitivity and 100% specificity but often it is a balance. Above, neither is 100% but they are balanced (some FP and an equal amount of FN).

If we want to capture all cases, we have to move the cutoff value of the test to the left. This <u>will</u> result in more false positives.

MAXIMIZE SENSITIVITY

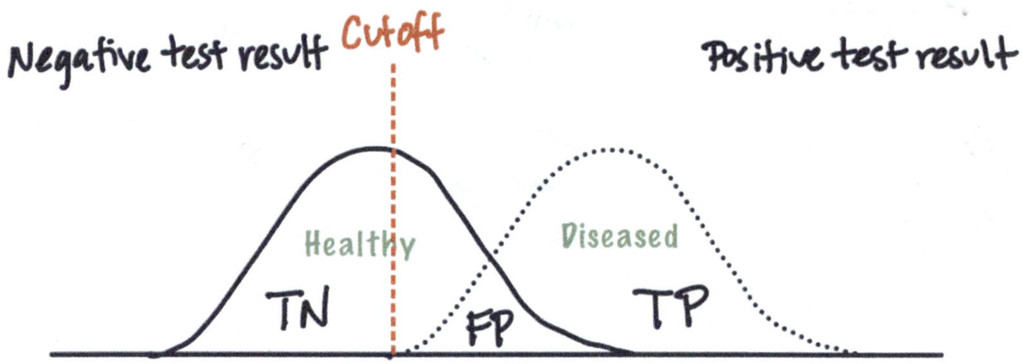

When might we want this?

We know some tests (Ex: rapid HIV) are going to have false positives. They are intended to help catch as many positives as possible so we back it up with a more accurate blood test on all positives from rapid testing to better rule OUT the diagnosis.

If initial does minimal/no harm, maximize: pregnancy test, flu screen, uti screen.

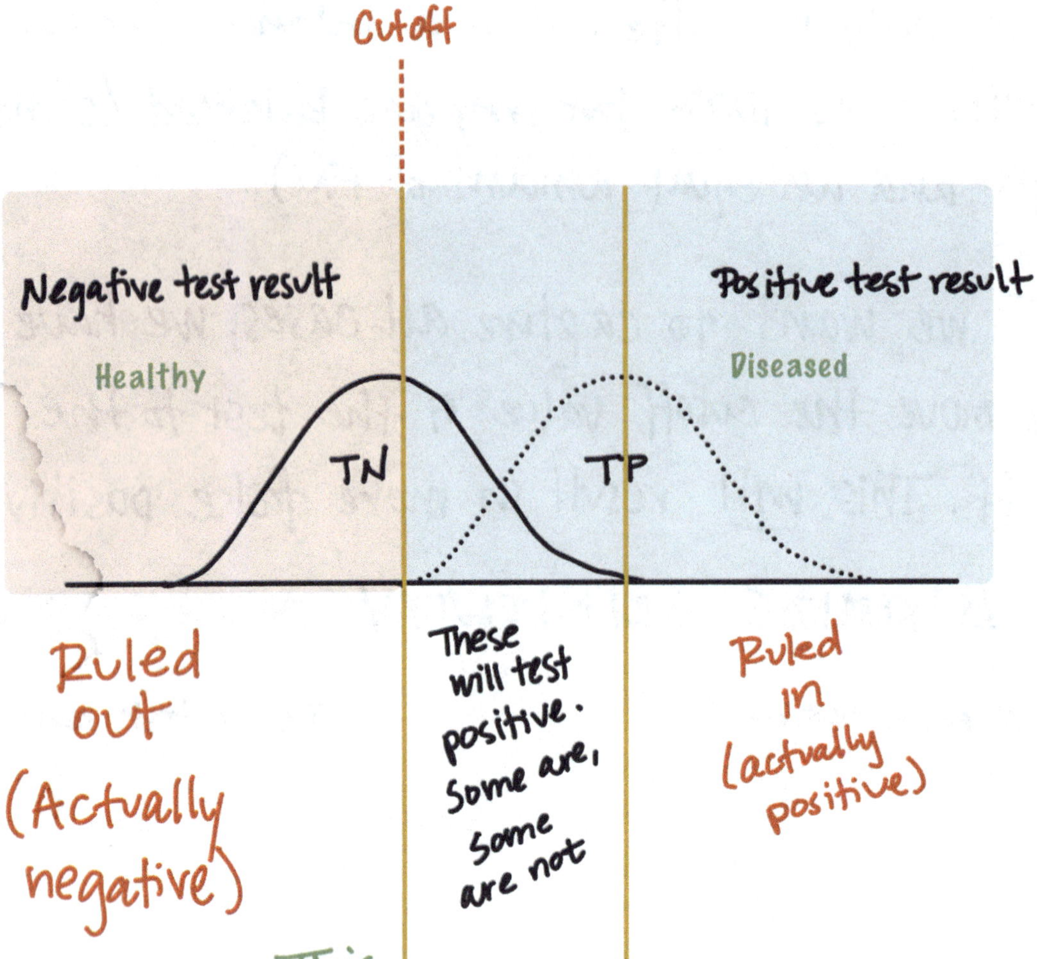

This line is 100% sensitivity

More important to correctly identify those with a concussion than determine they do not.

In this example, you only have false positives.

If + there is a chance you are −.
If − you are definitely −. SNOUT

MAXIMIZE SPECIFICITY

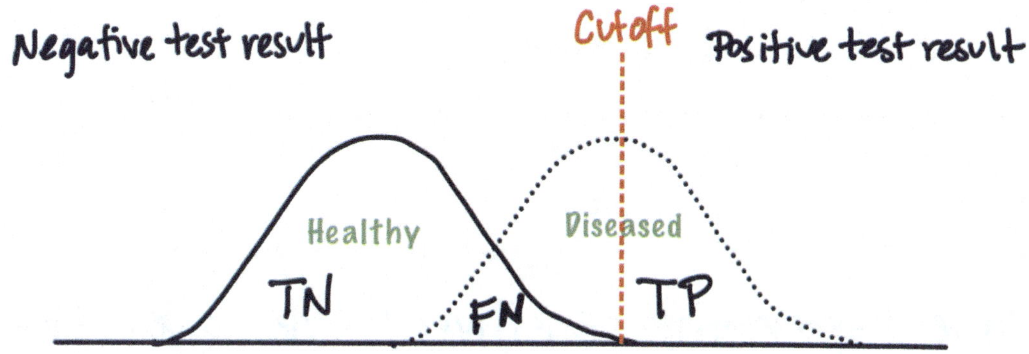

When might we want this?

Sometimes it is very important to be definitive that someone does have a disease or outcome, for example a fatal disease or Syphilis when pregnant. In these cases, a false positive test could cause more harm than good so we maximize our ability to rule disease IN.

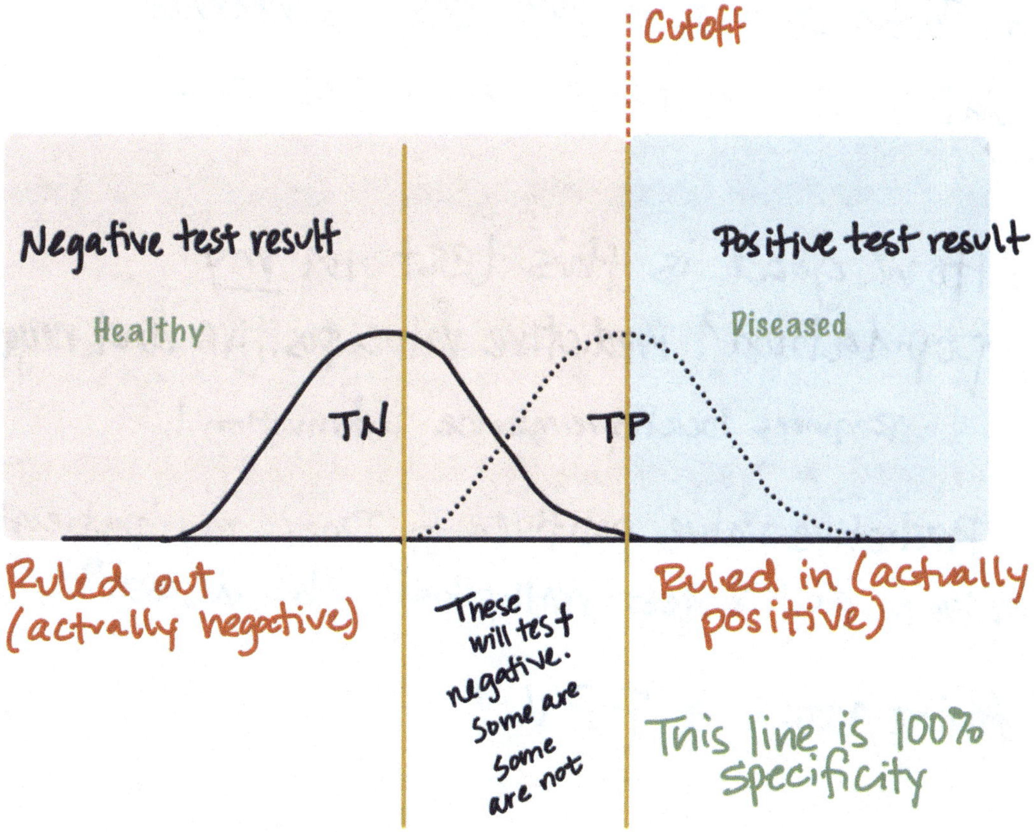

In this example, you only have false negatives.

If − there is a chance you are +.
If + you are definitely +. SPIN

The higher the sensitivity, the lower the specificity.

The higher the specificity, the lower the sensitivity.

If both are low, the test is neither valid nor reliable → do not use.

B) How good is this test in <u>my</u> population? Predictive value positive and negative

Requires local prevalence information!

1) Predictive value positive − Does my patient with a positive test really have the disease?

Abbreviated → PPV

Gold Standard

New Test	+	−
+	TP A	FP B
−	FN C	TN D

$$PPV = \frac{TP}{TP+FP}$$

Also seen as

$$\frac{A}{A+B}$$

If specificity increases, so does PPV because TN increases

2) Negative predictive value — Does my patient with a negative test really not have the disease?

Abbreviated → NPV

Gold Standard

New Test	+	−
+	TP A	FP B
−	FN C	TN D

$$NPV = \frac{TN}{TN+FN}$$

Also seen as

$$\frac{D}{C+D}$$

If prevalence is high] PPV is high
NPV is low

If prevalence is low] PPV is low
NPV is high

Example 1: You have 1000 patients and a local prevalence of 0%. The sensitivity of your test is 80% and the specificity is 87%.

1000 x 0% = 0 patients with the disease = A+C

1000 − 0 = 1000 patients without the disease = B+D

1000 x .87 (specificity) = 870 people are true negatives

$$\text{Specificity} = \frac{TN}{TN+FP} \quad .87 = \frac{x}{1000} = 870 \text{ TN}$$

Total − TN = 1000 − 870 = 130 = FP

Gold standard → reliable <u>and</u> valid

Other test or tool	+	−	Total
+	0	130	130
−	0	870	870
Total	0	1000	1000

PPV = A / A+B = $\frac{0}{130}$ = 0 → 0%

NPV = D / C+D = $\frac{870}{870}$ = 1 → 100%

If sensitivity is 80% and specificity is 87%

If prevalence	0%	10%	80%	100%
PPV	0%			100%
NPV	100%			0%

If the opposite were true and the prevalence was 100%

Example 2: You have 1000 patients and local prevalence is 10%. The sensitivity is 80% and the specificity is 87%.

1000 x 10% = 100 patients with the disease = A + C

1000 − 100 = 900 patients without the disease = B + D

900 x .87 (specificity) = 783 people are true negatives

900 − 783 = 117 = FP

Your test correctly identified 783 negative patients but missed 117 negative patients.

Gold standard → reliable and valid

Other test or tool	+	−	
+	80	117	197
−	20	783	803
	100	900	1000

You know the sensitivity is 80%.

$100 \times .80 = 80 = TP$

$100 - 80 = 20 = FN$

Your test correctly identified 80 positive patients but missed 20 positive patients.

$$PPV = A/A{+}B = \frac{80}{80+117} = \frac{80}{197} = .41 \qquad 41\%$$

$$NPV = D/C{+}D = \frac{783}{20+783} = \frac{783}{803} = .98 \qquad 98\%$$

If sensitivity is 80% and specificity is 87%

If prevalence	0%	10%	80%	100%
PPV	0%	41%		100%
NPV	100%	98%		0%

Example 3: You have 1000 patients and local prevalence is 80%. The sensitivity is 80% and the specificity is 87%.

1000 x 80% = 800 patients with the disease = A+C

1000 − 800 = 200 patients without the disease = B+D

200 x .87 (specificity) = 174 people are true negatives

200 − 174 = 26 = FP

Your test correctly identified 174 negative patients but missed 26 negative patients.

Gold standard → reliable and valid

Other test or tool		+	−	
	+		26	
	−		174	
		800	200	1000

You know the sensitivity is 80%

800 x .80 = 640 = TP

800 − 640 = 160 = FN

Your test correctly identified 640 positive patients but missed 160 positive patients.

Gold standard → reliable and valid

Other test or tool	+	−	
+	640	26	666
−	160	174	334
	800	200	1000

$$PPV = A/A+B = \frac{640}{666} = .96$$

96%

$$NPV = D/C+D = \frac{174}{334} = .52$$

52%

If sensitivity is 80% and specificity is 87%

If prevalence	0%	10%	80%	100%
PPV	0%	41%	96%	100%
NPV	100%	98%	52%	0%

Made in the USA
Monee, IL
03 January 2025

75899662R00096